MARVELOUS WAY OF NEEDLES

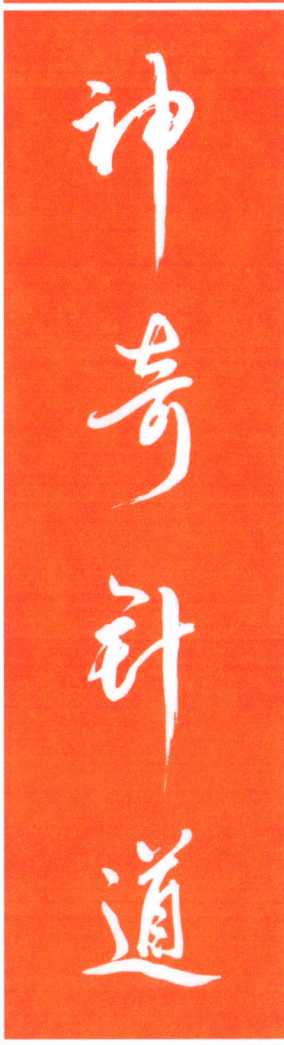

神奇針道

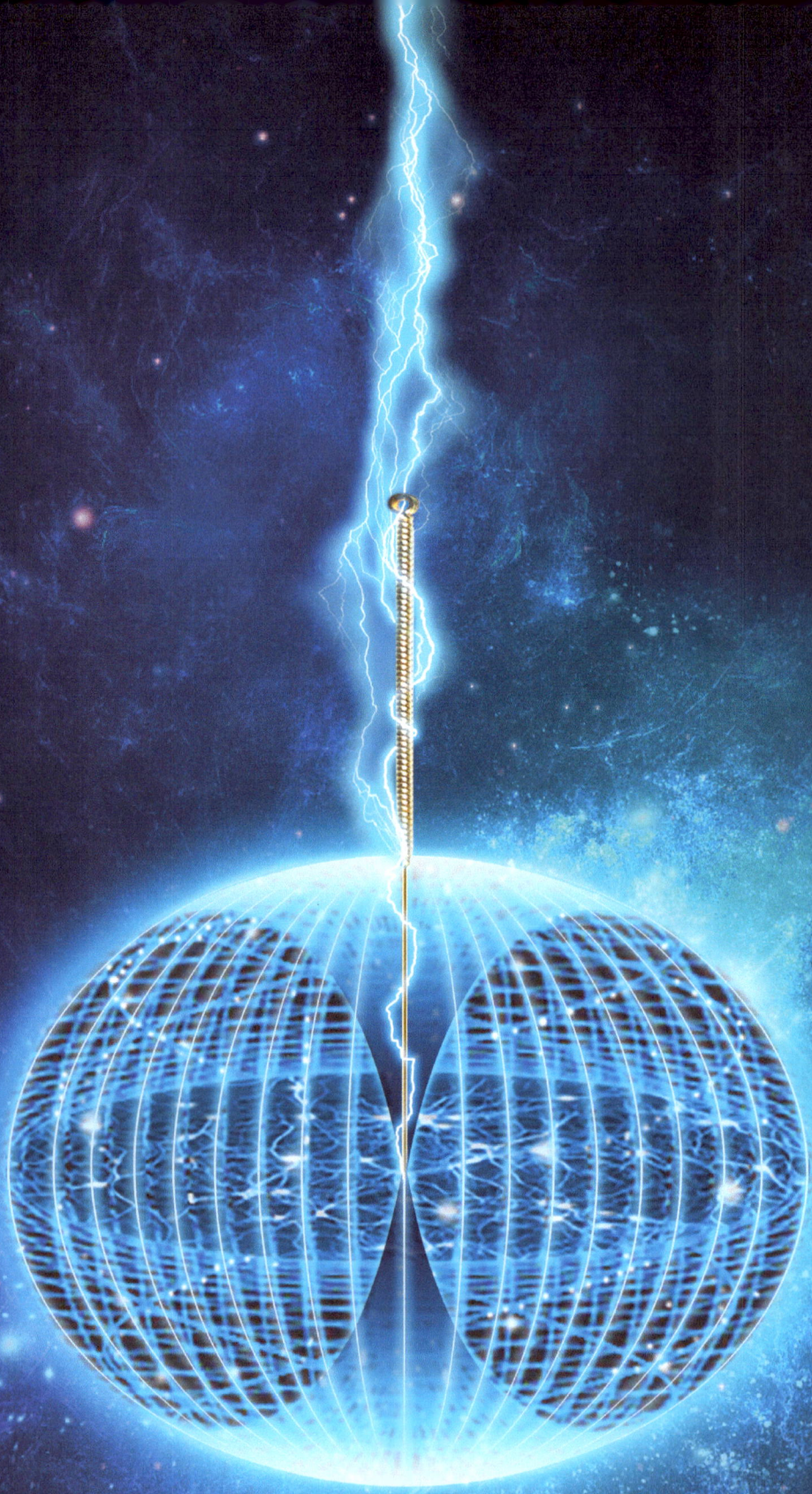

The inferior doctor only knows how to perform acupuncture on a particular acupoint. The superior doctor knows that to maximize treatment he must not only needle the point but stimulate the Ji gate as well. It could even be said that in the hands of a superior doctor the needle is connected to a higher phenomenon which for lack of a better term we can call the Divine Matrix. An earthly comparison could be made to the way your cell phone is invisibly connected to the Internet via wi fi.

MARVELOUS
Way of
NEEDLES

Reading Ling Shu Nine Needles
and Twelve Yuan-Source Points

Dr. Jiao Shun Fa

Translation

Dr. Tsoi Nam Chan

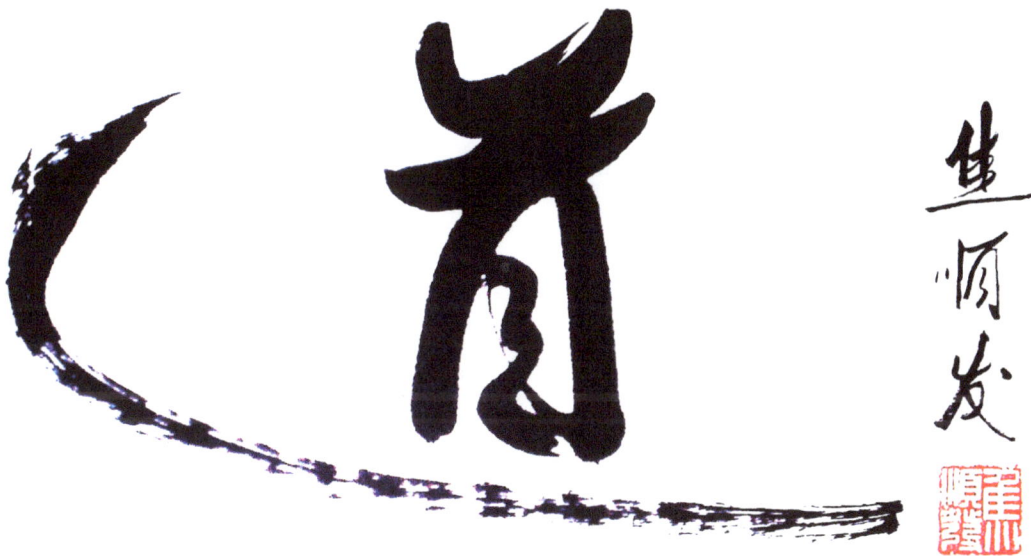

"DAO"
Calligraphy by Dr. Jiao

1st edition published by U.N. Acupuncture Center in 2019
307 E 44th Street, NYC, NY 10017, USA
Medicalmidtown@gmail.com

Disclaimer

Art, design and editing: Dr. Tsoi Nam Chan
Calligraphy: Dr. Jiao Shun Fa
Computer Graphic: Cindy X.W. Feng
Special thanks: my mother and father; my brothers Shek Man, Chor Man,
Kwok Wai, Kwok Hung, Yau Nam, Hoo *Sang* and my sister Yuet Sheung
Thanks also to: Lucy Yu, and Sabrina Seid

ISBN:
Printed in New York, USA

Foreword

Marvelous Way of Needles

This pioneering work offers readers an entirely new interpretation of acupuncture's *Jing-mai* theories, as postulated by Dr. Jiao Shun Fa. Dr. Jiao's work is based on ancient texts from the famous Chinese text, *The Yellow Emperor's Inner Canon*, as well as on 40 years experience developing clinical acupuncture treatments and conducting extensive medical research in the field of Chinese medicine. His medical writings include Head Acupuncture, Jiao Shun Fa *Head Acupuncture, Carotid Drip Liquid in the Treatment of Cerebrovascular Disease, Seeking the Truth of Chinese Acupuncture and Moxibustion, Soul of Chinese Acupuncture and Moxibustion, Acupuncture and Moxibustion Theory and Clinical Practice, Treating Diseases with Acupuncture* and more than ten other texts published in China and abroad. This new version of the classic Chinese medical text, the *Ling Shu - Nine Needles and Twelve Yuan-Source Points*, is his latest work and in many ways his most important contribution to the literature of contemporary Chinese medicine.

Acupuncture treatment is an ancient healing science developed by scholars millennia ago in ancient China. As early as 2500 B.C., its fundamental method of treating disease by inserting needles into key energy points throughout the body was explained in the first chapter of the *Ling Shu*. This groundbreaking book has remained a classic of Chinese medicine since the time it was written. Yet, due to misunderstandings of its sophisticated and complex content over the centuries, a substantial part of the *Ling Shu's* essential teachings has been lost or misinterpreted. This loss, in turn, has had a profoundly negative impact on the transmission of accurate acupuncture knowledge, even up to the present day.

The time has come, therefore, for a new interpretation of this ancient text – an interpretation that revises the many errors and misinterpretations that have plagued this great work over the centuries, and that better captures its original meaning and intent. The present book, it is hoped, will provide this needed corrective, amending errors that have crept into the text, clarifying important medical issues, and presenting its luminous medical insights for the use of future generations to come.

By <u>Dr. Tsoi Nam Chan</u>

Introduction

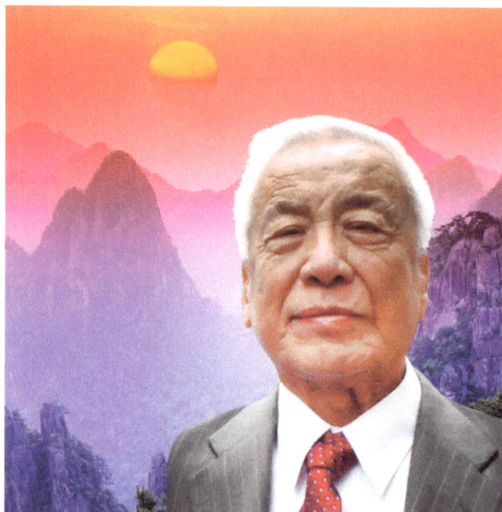

Dr. Jiao Shun Fa was born on December 25, 1938 in High Canal Village, *Ji*shan County, West Commune in Shanxi province, China. He currently serves as professor and chief physician, where he is a member of the China Association of Acupuncture and Moxibustion, and Chairman of the Acupuncture and Moxibustion Society in Shanxi province.

In 1970 Jiao Shun Fa invented "head acupuncture," a medical protocol that has been used successfully over the past several decades to treat a variety of brain disorders. In 1976, he developed a new treatment for cerebral vascular disease using carotid artery medicinal drips. Over the years, Dr. Jiao has promoted this method and its application throughout China. In 1986, he received a first prize National Award for his work in the field and for significant achievements in the development of Chinese medicine.

Dr. Jiao has worked tirelessly for more than 40 years developing clinical acupuncture treatments and conducting extensive medical research in the field of Chinese medicine. His medical writings include Head Acupuncture, Jiao Shun Fa *Head Acupuncture, Carotid Drip Liquid in the Treatment of Cerebrovascular Disease, Seeking the Truth of Chinese Acupuncture and Moxibustion, Soul of Chinese Acupuncture and Moxibustion, Acupuncture and Moxibustion Theory and Clinical Practice, Treating Diseases with Acupuncture,* and more than ten other texts published in China and abroad. His new version of the classic Chinese medical text, the *Ling Shu,* is his latest and in many ways most important contribution to the literature of contemporary Chinese medicine.

Preface

Though I have read *Nine Needles and Twelve Source Points* for more than 40 years, each time I delve into its profound writings I experience yet another new inspiration. One needs not only a calm mind and clear thoughts to read this text but also a capacity for bold decision making and a courageous initiative. Yet even now after all these years I make no claim to understanding this ancient text fully or to having plumbed its depths. At best I have formed a group of personal opinions about its teachings and have gained insights simply by being in daily contact with its wisdom. There is a saying in Chinese that speaks of "throwing bricks to attract jade." In other words, sometimes even an incomplete and imperfect attempt serves to help and motivate others. That is my intention with this present translation.

Jiao Shun Fa
October 30, 2007

One needs not only a calm and clear mind to read *Nine Needles and Twelve Source Points* but also boldness in decision making and courage to take initiative.

Jiao Shun Fa
February 27, 2007

Ling Shu Chapter 1- Nine Needles and Twelve Source Points sums up in depth research, core experiences and theoretical achievements of Chinese medical specialists in the treatment of disease with acupuncture over thousands of years. It advocates and promotes the treatment of disease by needling the *Jingmai*, and should be considered an advanced medical science for its rational theories, excellent methods, and unique therapeutic effects.

Jiao Shun Fa
March 18, 2007

Prologue

Acupuncture treatment is an ancient healing science that was developed by scholars millenia ago in ancient China. As early as 2500 B.C., its fundamental method of treating disease by inserting needles into key energy points throughout the body was explained in the first chapter of the famous *Ling Shu - Nine Needles and Twelve Yuan-Source Points*. This groundbreaking book has remained a classic in Chinese medicine since the time it was written.

However, due to misunderstandings of its sophisticated and complex content over the centuries, a substantial part of the *Ling Shu*'s essential teachings has been lost or misinterpreted. This loss, in turn, has had a profoundly negative impact on the transmission of accurate acupuncture knowledge, even up to the present day.

The time has come, therefore, for a new interpretation of this ancient text – an interpretation that revises the many errors and misinterpretations that have plagued this great work over the centuries, and that better captures its original meaning and intent.

The present book, it is hoped, will provide this needed corrective, amending errors that have crept into the text, clarifying important medical issues, and presenting its luminous medical insights for the use of future generations to come.

Jiao Shun Fa
February 24, 2008

Table of Content

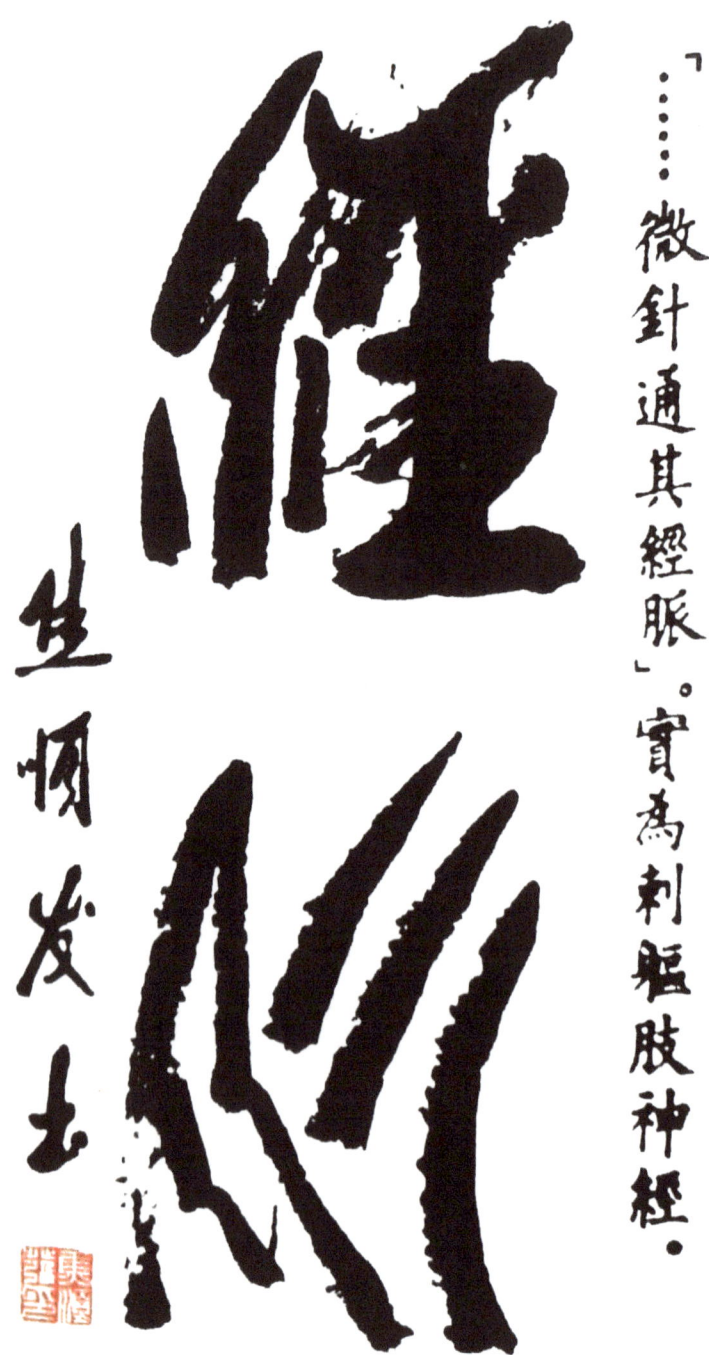

「……微針通其經脈」。實為刺軀肢神經。

生恆發書

"*JINGMAI*"
Calligraphy by Dr. Jiao

CHAPTER ONE

Original Text - Summary of Notes

"*A poor doctor knows only the physical location of an acu-point, while a superior doctor seeks the spirit (Shen) (inside the point). This spirit is wondrous; it is like a distinguished guest in the door.*"

Section 1 - Summary of the Original Text

1 - Original Text: "The Yellow Emperor said to *Qi* Bo: I treat my people as if they were my own children. I feed them and collect land taxes from them. I have pity on their inability to take care of their own health and on their vulnerability to diseases. I want to protect them from being treated by (harsh) drugs or stone implements that may cause side effects and pain. To accomplish this feat I prefer to use fine needles that can be inserted into the skin. These needles activate the *Jingmai* (acupuncture meridians), regulate and nourish the *Qi* (life force) and blood, manage the currents and counter currents (of energy), and assemble the entering/exiting convergent points. This system of fine needle acupuncture can certainly be passed down to future generations and last forever. Still, it must adhere to a set of clear rules. It must be easy to use, difficult to forget, and become a classical doctrine. We must, therefore, summarize its teachings into chapters, clarify what is extrinsic in it and what is intrinsic, and define both an end and a beginning. In short, in order to make everything appear organized, we must create a book titled 'Acupuncture doctrine.' I would like to hear your opinion on this matter."

Summary of Notes: The Yellow Emperor explained to *Qi* Bo that people cannot afford the taxes they must pay due to illness. He wants to protect them from drug or stone implement treatment, and encourages the use of fine needles that pierce the *Jingmais* (that is, pierce the somatic nerves), thus regulating *Qi* and curing disease. [Please refer to Note 1 and 2 in Chapter 1, Section 1.2]

This method of treatment can definitely be transmitted to future generations, but legislation (organization) is necessary. You should, therefore, write a book termed "Acupuncture Doctrine." Divide this book into the following chapters: diagnosis of major illness, *Jingmai*, the distribution of nerves in the visceras and body surface, acupuncture methods, and principles of point selection. Write all this information down in true, simple language that makes the book easy to use and difficult to forget. This information will then be passed down from generation to generation, lasting for numberless years without cease. I would like to hear your views on this subject.

2 - Original Text: "A poor doctor knows only the physical location of an acupoint, while a superior doctor seeks the spirit (*Shen*) (inside the point). This spirit is wondrous; it is like a distinguished guest in the door."

Summary of Notes: An inferior doctor's only concern is which physical location on the body to perform acupuncture. A superior doctor knows how, when and where to needle the *Shen* point. *Shen* is very wondrous, like a distinguished guest in the door. *Shen* is described here. Refer specifically to the *Jingmai* within the acupoint - the body somatic nerves. Please refer to Note 3 in Chapter 1, Section 1.2.

T.N. Chan Interpretation: It could be that the needle is connected to the divine matrix.

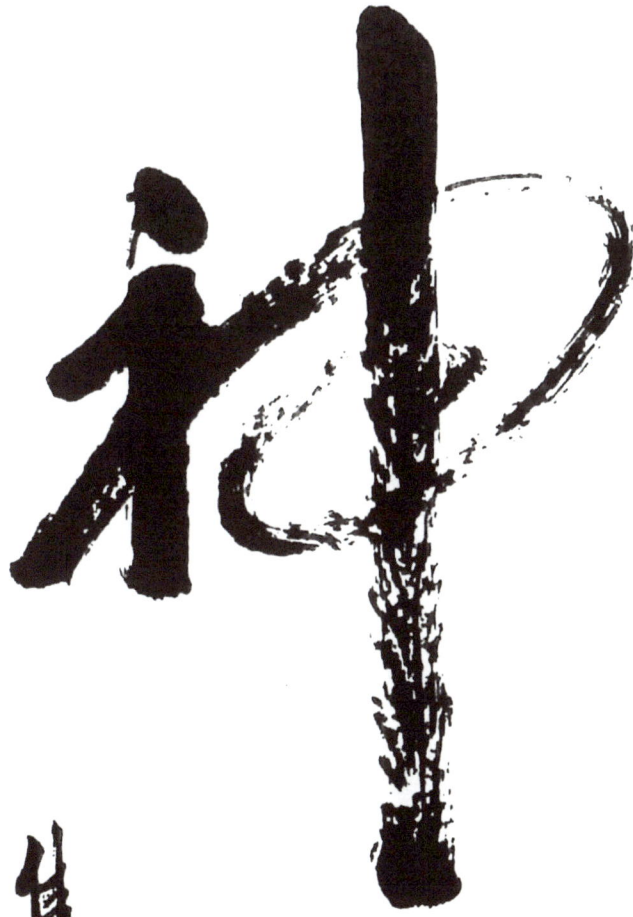

神

焦顺发

「......守神」。特
指守經脈，實
為刺軀肢神經。

"SHEN"
Calligraphy by Dr. Jiao

3 - Original Text: "A poor doctor only knows how to look for the physical joints (*Guan*) while the superior doctor knows how to find *Ji* – gate mechanism in the point. The movement of *Ji* never exceeds its space. When we observe it from the outside *Ji* activity appears tranquil in the space it occupies. It appears to have only a slight movement. Its coming cannot be met and its going cannot be followed or grasped. Those who understand the gate mechanism are able to pierce the points precisely without missing a hair's breadth. Those who do not understand gate mechanism will miss the timing of *Qi*. Piercing points in a random way is useless. Knowing where *Qi* is coming from and where it is going and timing of *Qi* to get the best result is important. This phenomenon is really wondrous. The poor doctor remains in the dark (about it), while the superior doctor knows all these (important facts)."

Summary of Notes: Poor doctors only know how to perform acupuncture on the physical location of the points, while superior doctors know how to needle the gate, *Ji*. The *Ji* is located in the point itself, and its *Ji* activity at this point never exceeds its space. Through anatomical and physiological studies, they have found in the point of *Ji* that the surface appears outwardly tranquil with only slight pulsation. But in reality, information is being rapidly conveyed (in and out) of the *Ji*. Most doctors may not experience this fact through commonly used methods. By understanding the vital timing of the *Ji*, gate mechanism, it will be easy to pierce the target (reach the heart of the point). Not knowing the vital timing of the *Ji* mechanism is the same as locking the trigger (of a gun). Shooting will not be possible, and such random piercing is not going to hit the target. Poor doctors are in the dark about these principles, while superior doctors possess unique skills and can induce this wondrous phenomenon. Please refer to Note 4 in Chapter 1, Section 1.2.

4 - Original Text: "The term 'going' means 'counter flow.' The term 'coming' means to 'follow.' By knowing 'counter flow' and 'follow,' a doctor can perform acupuncture without asking (needless questions). *Qi* activity is not made deficient by withdrawing the needle with the tip going against the pathway of the *Jingmai*, and is not in excess by following the flow of the *Jingmai* with the needles. Counter flow and follow: if you understand this theory you definitely have mastered the great art of needling technique."

Summary of Notes: When applying acupuncture, the direction of needling that diminishes the "arrival of *Qi*" is described as "the direction of counter flow," while the direction that triggers the "arrival of *Qi*" is called "flow." By knowing the meaning of flow and counter flow you can insert the needle (without fear). Withdrawing the needle, the "arrival of *Qi*" will then be reduced; thrusting it during the "arrival of *Qi*" enhances it. Follow your instinct to regulate the intensity of *Qi* by moving the needle backwards and forward. This is the most important technique in clinical acupuncture.

5 - Original Text: "Deficiency by filling, excess by draining, chronic stagnation by eliminating, and over abundance of evil *Qi* by withdrawing."

Summary of Notes: For "deficiency by filling," one needs to needle the points repeatedly to promote *Qi* activity until signs of activity are obvious. This method is called "excess." Needling should stop when the *Jingmai* is activated. For "excess by draining" one should withdraw the needle a bit to relax the intensity of *Qi* activity. For "chronic stagnation by eliminating" the doctor must withdraw the needle slightly when it meets resistance and cannot be fully inserted, then change its direction. "Over abundance of evil *Qi* by withdrawing" refers to the process of pulling back the needle when there is obvious pain in order to stop unpleasant sensations. Please refer to Note 5 in Chapter 1, Section 1.2.

6 - Original Text: "*The Great Essentials* says: 'Slow, then rapid is excess. Rapid, then excess is deficiency. Speaking of excess and deficiency, sometimes it is there, sometimes it is not. As for examining before and after, sometimes it is there, sometimes it is not. Speaking of the feeling of empty and full, sometimes we gain it and sometimes we lose it.'"

Summary of Notes: This is an old text from ancient times. "Slow then rapid is excess" means that when the tip of the acupuncture needle reaches the correct depth of the *Jingmai*, push it in slowly. If *Qi* appears immediately, the needle tip is considered to be at the solids level. This "solidness" demonstrates that contact has been made with the *Jingmai* or somatic nerves. "Rapid then slow is empty" means that despite the fact that the piercing speed is fast and hard the *Qi* does not arrive. This means that the needle is still in the state of "emptiness" (that is, it has not yet pierced *Jingmai*), a condition that is referred to as "empty." Sometimes it is there, sometimes it is not." This phrase means that when needling *Jingmai* the solidness and emptiness that we talked about is sometimes there, while at other times it cannot be felt. When observing and comparing the situation before and after the arrival of *Qi*, sometimes there is sensation and sometimes there is no sensation. In reference to excess and deficiency, sometimes it is there, sometimes it is not there. That is to say, with emptiness and solidness, sometimes there is sensation and sometimes there is no sensation. Please refer to Note 6 in Chapter 1, Section 1.2.

7 - Original Text: "Needling precisely has to do with being quick and being slow."

Summary of Notes: Experienced doctors are able to contact the *Jingmai* (somatic nerves) and trigger the arrival of *Qi* very quickly. It is more difficult for poor doctors to pierce and hit the *Jingmai* in this way. The difference between the two is whether or not they can quickly trigger the arrival of *Qi*.

8 - Original Text: "To drain is called Ying. The meaning of Ying is to hold it inside, release and expel the Evil *Qi*, discharge Yang, and then remove the needle. Evil *Qi* can be drained in this way. To tonify is to follow. The sensation of following is as if to forget, to stimulate and press like a mosquito or gadfly bite, to detain and return, then to withdraw like an arrow leaving the bowstring. Command the left to follow the right; this will cause the *Qi* to stop."

Summary of Notes: Dispersion is called Ying. This means that to disperse you must have Ying energy present. The meaning of Ying is to push the needle into the acupoint and then insert it forward. When the sign of *Qi* arrival suddenly appears the patient often cannot stand the pain. At this point, you pull the needle backwards and the *Qi* arrival sensation will diminish or disappear.

To tonify is to follow. This means that to tonify one must push the needle into the acupoint. This specific technique calls for needling the acupoint, and piercing close to the *Jingmai* (somatic nerves) or when the tip of the needle is getting close to its surface. When the *Qi* has arrived, however, (the situation) is still not ideal and there is still need to tonify, to push the needle slowly inward. Be cautious here, stopping as soon as it is obvious that the *Qi* is reached. If the needle is pushed too quickly or forcefully, or if the direction is changed, the arrival of *Qi* may disappear entirely.

9 – Original Text: "As for the way to hold a needle, holding it tight is precious. Therefore, hold the needle straight and pierce perpendicularly. Do not needle to the left or right. Observe attentively. Watch the patient (carefully) while you work."

Summary of Notes: Hold the needle tightly and insert it perpendicularly. Observe closely. The arrival of *Qi Ji* proves that the needle has reached the *Jingmai* (the somatic nerve). At this point stop needling immediately.

10 - Original Text: "Piercing and *Qi* has not arrived. Don't ask how many times; pierce and *Qi* arrives, then remove the needle and no more piercing."

Summary of Notes: When using fine needles to pierce *Jingmai*, if there is no sign of *Qi Ji* appearing, do not worry about how many times you pierce. Simply continue piercing until *Qi Ji* arrives, then remove the needle and stop. Please refer to Note 7 in Chapter 1, Section 1.2.

11 - Original Text: "The essence of needling is that once *Qi* arrives a (healing) effect is generated. This effect appears quickly, as when the wind blows away the clouds, suddenly causing the sky to become clear and blue. This process describes the complete *Tao* of needling."

Summary of Notes: During acupuncture, as soon as *Qi* becomes active the therapeutic effect is obtained. This effect comes quickly, as when the wind suddenly blows away the dark clouds. Please refer to Note 8 in Chapter 1, Section 1.2.

12 - Original Text: "The Yellow Emperor said, 'I would like to know about the origins of the five *Zang* and six *Fu* organs.' *Qi* Bo replied, "Five *Zang*, Five *Shu*, five times five is 25 *Shu*. Six *Fu* and six *Shu*, six times six is 36 *Shu*. Twelve *Jingmai* and 15 *Luo Mai* constitute the 27 *Qi* pathways on which the *Qi* travels up and down. Where *Qi* comes out it is called *Jing* (the well) point, where it trickles it is called Ying (the spring) point, when it is poured it is called *Shu* (the stream) point. Where it runs it is called *Jing* (the river) point, and when it gathers it is called He (the lake) point. The 27 *Qi* pathways all depend on these five *Shu* points. Crossings of *Jie*, 365 junctions. For those who know the essence, one sentence is enough; those who do not know talk pointlessly and endlessly. The so-called *Jie* are places where *Shen Qi* travels in and out; they are not skin, muscles, tendons and bones.'"

Summary of Notes: The Yellow Emperor said he wished to know the origins of the five *Zang* and six *Fu* organs. *Qi* Bo said that the five *Zang* organs each have five *Shu* points. There is a total of 25 *Shu* points. Six *Zang* organs each have six *Shu* points making a total of 36 *Shu* points. There are 12 *Jingmai*, and 15 *Luo Mai*. The *Jing Qi* all have to go through the five *Shu* points.

In conclusion, he said "Crossings of *Jie*, 365 hui" means that the 365 points throughout the body are formed by junctions of *Jingmai* that cross each other many times. This knowledge is the result of scientific research done long ago. But (through the years) there have been different interpretations of this principle and experts have not been able to agree. So people say that "for those who know the essence, one sentence is enough; those who do not know talk pointlessly and endlessly." In modern times, the superior doctor summarizes the meaning of *Jie* in one statement, proclaiming that "*Jie* are junctions of the anterolateral and posterolateral spinal tracts and neurofilaments that cross multiple times. These junctions freely transmit (motional and sensory) information, and they are neither skin, muscles, tendons nor bones." Please refer to Note 9 in Chapter 1, Section 1.2.

13 - Original Text: "Observe the eyes; one can know (much from) their dilation and recovery."

Summary of Notes: By examining the size of the pupils, their shape, and their sensitivity to light, one can judge the condition of the patient. Please refer to Note 10 in Chapter 1, Section 1.2.

14 - Original Text: "Whenever one starts to practice acupuncture, one must check the patient's pulse, examine the condition of the patient's *Qi*, and then begin treatment."

Summary of Notes: Whenever doctors start to do acupuncture they must check the pulse to gauge the condition of the patient and confirm whether or not acupuncture is a suitable healing method for this particular disease.

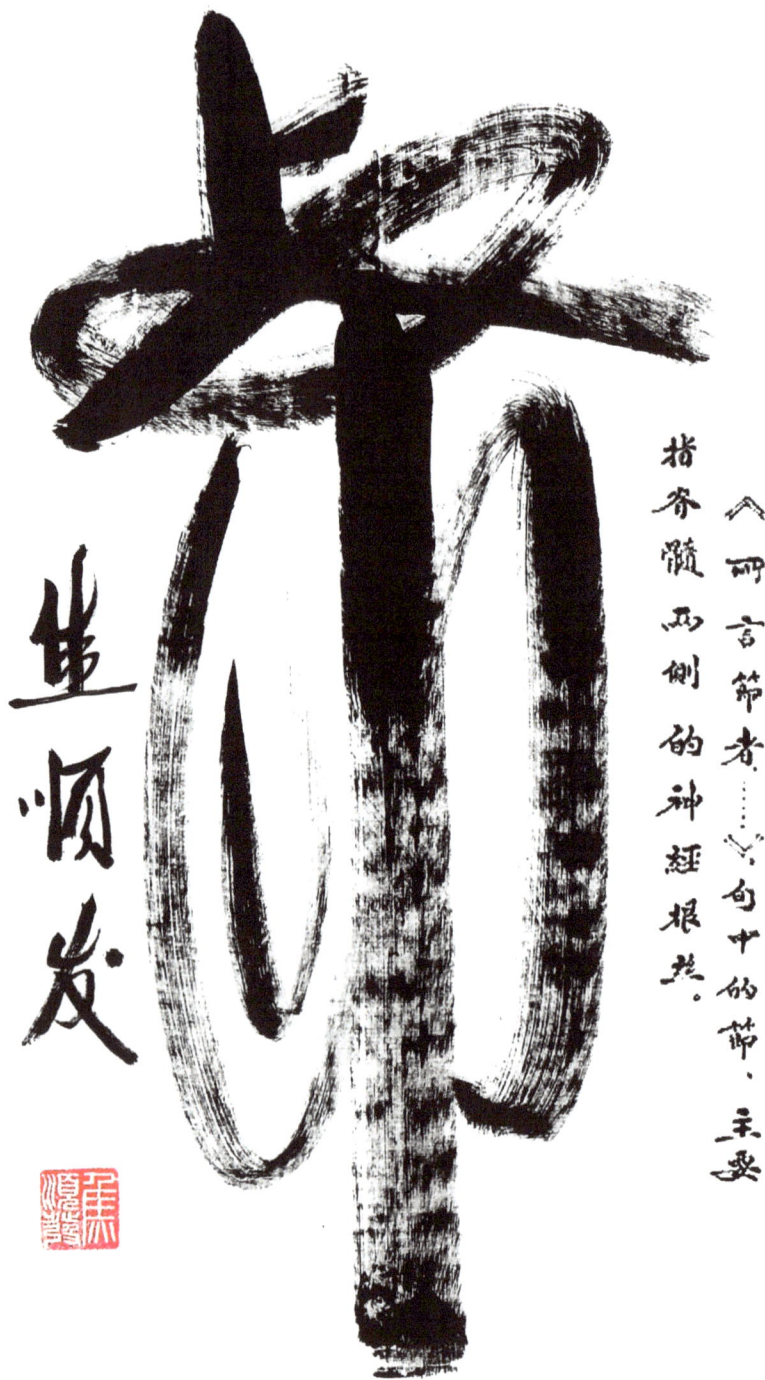

崔顺发

《矾言節者……》句中的節，主要指脊髓两侧的神経根处。

"*DU JIE*"
Calligraphy by Dr. Jiao

15 - Original Text: "The five *Zang* and six *Fu* organs have 12 *Yuan*-source points. The 12 *Yuan*-source points originate from the four '*Guan*' (elbow and knee joints). The four '*Guan*' are used to treat diseases in the five *Zang* organs. When there is disease in the five *Zang* organs the 12 *Yuan*-source points should be chosen for treatment. The 12 *Yuan*-source points are the keys for the five *Zang* organs; (they help them) receive the *Qi* and the 'tastes' (essence) of the 365 *Jie* (points). When there is illness in one of the five *Zang* organs there will be reactions appearing in the 12 *Yuan* (source) points. The 12 source points have their outlet points (for these reactions) respectively. Knowing their source clearly and seeing their reactions, the doctor can identify disease in the five *Zang* organs. For the lung, the *Yuan*-source point is originated from LU 9 (*tài yuān*). For the heart, the *Yuan* point is from PC 7 (*dà lín*). That of liver is at LV 3 (*tài chōng*). That of spleen is at SP 3 (*tài bái*). That of kidney is at KI 3 (*tài xī*). That of Gao is at RN 15 (*jiū wěi*), and that of the *Huang* is at RN 6 (*qì hǎi*). All of these 12 source points (are used to) treat the diseases of the five *Zang* and the six *Fu* organs of the body."

Summary of Notes: There are five *Zang* and six *Fu* organs. The six *Fu* have 12 source points. Although those 12 source points are located at the end of the body's four limbs, they are nonetheless connected to the five *Zang* and six *Fu*. Therefore, when there is disease in the *Zang* and *Fu* organs, the 12 source points should be chosen for treatment. These 12 source points have their origins respectively. The *Yuan*-source point of the lung is originated from from LU 9 (*tài yuān*), that of heart is from PC 7 (*dà líng*), that of liver is from LV 3 (*tài chōng*)… that of spleen is from SP 3 (*tài bái*), that of kidney is from KI 3 (*tài xī*), that of the Gao is from RN 15 (*jiū wěi*), and that of the *Huang* is from RN 6 (*qì hǎi*). All of these 12 source points are used treat the disease of the five *Zang* and the six *Fu* organs.

16 - Original Text: "Diseases of the five *Zang* organs are like thorns, dirty stains, knotted ropes or (dense) obstructions. (Yet), even thorns that nestle in the flesh for a long period of time can be pulled out. Even old stains can be cleaned. Even knots can be untied and obstructions cleared. It is wrong to believe that chronic diseases can never be cured. Those who are skillful at acupuncture can remove disease as if they were pulling out a thorn, cleaning a stain, opening a knot or clearing up blockages. Chronic diseases can be put to an end. People who say chronic diseases are incurable have not fully mastered the technique of using fine needles to pierce the *Jingmai*."

Summary of Notes: (Chronic) disease in the five *Zang* is like a thorn, a knot, or a flowing river that is partially or fully blocked. Even though a thorn has been in the skin for a long period of time, however, it can still be pulled out, just as old stains can be washed away, knots that have been tied for a long time can be loosened, and rivers that have long been blocked can be cleared. Some people say chronic disease cannot be cured. This notion is incorrect. The technique of using fine needles to pierce *Jingmai* (somatic nerves) can be used to treat chronic diseases just as a thorn can be pulled from the skin, a stain can be cleaned, and the blockades in a river removed. People who say chronic diseases are incurable have not fully mastered the technique of using fine needles to pierce *Jingmai* (somatic nerves).

Section 2 notes

I. Reflections on the first paragraph of *Ling Shu Chapter 1 – Nine Needles and Twelve Source Points.*

In *Ling Shu Chapter 1 - Nine Needles and Twelve Source Points*, the Yellow Emperor says to *Qi* Bo, "I treat my people as if they were my children, feed them and collect land taxes from them. I have pity on their inability to take care of their own health and their vulnerability to diseases. I want to protect them from (harsh or useless) treatment by means of drugs or stone implements which may bring about side effects and pain. I prefer to use fine needles that can be inserted into the skin to activate the *Jingmai* and regulate and nourish *Qi* and blood, and manage the junctions where *Qi* flow and counter flow exit and enter. The art of using fine needle acupuncture treatment can certainly be passed down to the future generations. It must be easy to use, difficult to forget, and (ultimately) become a classical doctrine. Summarize this information into chapters. Clarify the extrinsic and the intrinsic. Define an end and a beginning. In order to make everything appear organized, we should start to write a book called 'Acupuncture doctrine.' I would like to hear your opinion."

Medical scholars have attempted to interpret and apply this paragraph ever since it was first written. Most have come up with oversimplified interpretations, missed the mark concerning the passage's deep importance, and failed to demonstrate its true and original meaning. For the fact is that this paragraph is the single most important passage in the entire *Ling Shu*. Why? Because it explicitly defines the stimulation of the *Jingmai* with fine needles as the most scientific and effective method there is for treating disease. The author of *Ling Shu* hoped that this system would last a long time and be widely applied by later generations to come.

This opening paragraph is thus not only marvelous and unique, but is highly sophisticated and thoroughly scientific. It should be regarded as the main principle of the *Ling Shu* and viewed as the core and soul of all acupuncture practice and theory. In short, this passage describes thoroughly and superbly the treatment of disease by needling the *Jingmais*. It succinctly cuts through all mystery (and obscurity), leaving informed readers in awe.

"I prefer to use fine needles that can be inserted into the skin to activate *Jingmai* and regulate and nourish *Qi* and blood, manage the junctions where *Qi* flow and counter flow, exit and enter." This sentence should be considered the core message of this first paragraph.

Approximately 5,000 years ago, Chinese medical experts began to explore methods of needling the trunk and extremities in order to treat disease. In these early days doctors used thick needles to penetrate tissue and even the vital organs. They found that by needling the trunk and extremities they could sometimes bring about healing, an effect that was likely related to the fact that their needles occasionally (and accidentaly) stimulated the *Jingmai*. This random method, however, frequently caused serious injury to patients and even death. The Treatise on Needling Contraindications was thus intentionally included in *Huang* Di Nei *Jing*-Su Wen to warn doctors against needing important organs and tissues, and to urge them to use fine rather than thick needles in their clincal practice.

Using fine needles to activate the *Jingmai* is a wonderful and unique method for treating disease. The idea that doctors should use such needles in acupuncture was an innovation, a kind of technological revolution. Fine needles themselves are very mysterious. *Nine Needles and Twelve Source Points* describes the point of the fine needle as being similar to the stinger of a mosquito. It also describes the tip of a fine needle as being extremely thin, almost too small to be seen with the naked eye. Millennia ago, when people first started practicing acupuncture, they used thick needles in various shapes and sizes, some quite large and ungainly. Through years of clinical practice the advantages and disadvantages of different needles were tested, and fine needles eventually emerged as the safest and most efficient tool. Although there were several good reasons for using fine needles, the primary benefit was that they could easily puncture the skin and stimulate the *Qi*, leading to a favorable therapeutic effect free from side effects. The doctors of the time settled on fine needles as an optimal tool to activate the *Jingmai*, and as the most effective and scientific method for treating disease.

The statement that needling "regulates *Qi* and blood" should be viewed as a significant discovery. "Regulate" refers to the regulatory functions that needles provide when needling the *Jingmais*. These functions include changes in the blood supply and increased *Qi* flow into the affected areas. This discovery not only revealed the principle behind treating disease but also showed that the body's *Jingmai* system exerts a powerful regulatory function on the whole body. Thus, people can maintain health by regulating their *Jingmai* systems and achieving a balance between the interior and exterior parts of the body. If the body is attacked by a disease, the disease can be completely cured by proper needling of the respective *Jingmai*.

"Manage its junction of flow and counter flow and entering/exiting points" is another profound scientific observation. Ying refers to managing the substances that nourish the body, as well as the *Jingamis* related to disease. Here, "*Shun ni chu ru zhi hui*" particularly refers to the somatic *Jingmais*. In terms of function they deliver information in and out; in terms of structure they cross many times, forming junction points.

As a result, it is known that the method of using fine needles to pierce *Jingmais* provides a scientific healing method that is mature and technologically advanced, a method that can be promoted and applied to resolve the health care problem of the people of China.

When we witness the discoveries that the ancients made 1800 years ago in the fields of neurology and physiology we learn that the *Jingmai* they identified were actually what modern science knows today as the somatic nerves. This means that as early as 2,500 years ago, when most of the world's medical knowledge was at a Stone Age level, Chinese medical experts were intimately familiar with the human nervous system, and were treating disease with a highly sophisticated system of needle stimulatiion and *Qi/* blood regulation.

"Can be pased down to the future generations" and "lasts forever." These definitive sentences tell us that the art of using fine needles to pierce the *Jingmai* is so effective that its techniques will be passed down from generation to generation, a prediction that has allready proven true many times over. Today, as a doctor who uses fine needles to treat disease in my own practice, I feel great warmth and excitement by reading these beautiful predictive sentences written 1800 years ago.

II. Reflections on "… I prefer to use fine needles to open up its *Jingmai*, to regulate its *Qi* and blood, and to manage its junctions where *Qi* flow and counter flow, exit and enter. To pass it down to future generations, it is necessary to set clear rules."

"I prefer to use fine needles to open up its *Jingmai*, to regulate its *Qi* and blood, and to manage its junctions where *Qi* flow and counter flow, exit and enter. To pass it down to future generations, it is necessary to set clear rules."

This passage, taken from the first paragraph of *Ling Shu - Nine Needles and Twelve Source Points* develops a master principle of Chinese medicine, and presents us with a very important and unusual concept indeed. At the time of its writing many Chinese physicians did not have a clear understanding of its meaning, and over the centuries this led to many difficulties and misunderstandings. As I reread these cogent and ground-breaking sentences today I feel a heartfelt surprise. The following are my thoughts on these writings. Feedback and advice on these thoughts from experts would be appreciated.

(A) Interpretation by most Chinese physicians:

Over the centuries many medical specialists attempted to interpret the content of the *Ling Shu* by explaining it in superficial ways and developing contradictory versions of its teachings. This is why people of subsequent generations slowly lost interest in the text, and why there is something of a prejudice against it even today among modern practitioners. Up until the present era the *Ling Shu* continues to remain misunderstood, unstudied, and ignored.

(B) My specific interpretations according to the doctrines:

a. "Thus, I prefer to use fine needles to open up the *Jingmai*" is a technical phrase concerning the treatment of disease. It refers to the art of using fine needles to pierce *Jingmai* and hence unblock *Jingmai Qi*. This quote effectively summarizes treatment methods used 2,500 years ago up till today.

b. Chinese medical experts have not reached a consensus on the ultimate meaning of *Jingmai*. There are various reasons for this lack of consensus, first among them being resistance to taking seriously the all important sentence: "wishing to use fine needles to activate *Jingmai*."

1. "Tiao *Qi Qi Xue*" - "Regulating *Qi* and blood"

The term "Regulating *Qi* and blood," represents a significant scientific breakthrough, especially as it relates to the use of acupuncture and *Jingmai* for treating disease. While scholars have agreed on this point, the key mechanism of the phrase has only been passed down through the years by oral transmission, since memorization and repetition are more common than intensive research.

2. "Manage its junctions where *Qi* flow and counter flow, exit and enter."

When deciphering the phrase "manage the junctions where *Qi* flows and counter flows, exit and enter" one should first understand the meaning of the abstruce term "junctions where *Qi* flows and counter flows, exit and enter." One should also understand why we use this term. When I first started to read this phrase almost 40 years ago I was completely lost. Years later I finally discovered that "junctions where *Qi* flow and counter flow, exit and enter" was by no means a casual description but was based on experience with anatomy, physiology and other scientific research, combined with deep thought and inspired deliberation.

Ling Shu includes separate chapters on the 12 *Jingmai*, the 12 *Jing Bie* (divergent *Jingmai*), and the 12 *Jin Jing* (the tendons and the muscular system that run along the *Jingmai*). Yet the authors of the *Nine Needles and Twelve Source Points* did not use the information from these chapters to describe the *Jingmai*. Why? Because they disagreed with the notion that the *Qi* of the 12 *Jingmai* travels in one direction. And so, based on conclusions reached from their own scientific research, they created the entirely new expression, "Junctions where *Qi* flows and counter flows, exits and enters" to describe the *Jingmai* as they understood it.

"Crossings of *Jie*, 365 junctions. For those who know the essence, one sentence is enough; those who do not know talk pointlessly and endlessly. The so-called '*Jie*' are places where *Shen Qi* travels in and out; they are not skin, muscles, tendons and bones."

I discovered that the above passage has a special relationship with the phrase "the junctions of counter flow, flow, exiting and entering points." In other words, we can say that "the junction of counterflow, flow, exiting and entering points" is a reference to

"Crossings of *Jie*, 365 junctions," and that "the so-called '*Jie*'" refers to where the *Shen Qi* (spirit energy) travels in and out.

Here it is necessary to be specific in clarifying the term "Crossings of *Jie*, 365 junctions." This sentence, we know, existed before the publication of *Ling Shu* (though the actual date of its writing cannot be verified). It was, however, clearly based on important findings made by ancient Chinese doctors during their anatomical researches on *Jingmai*. From an early date it was then applied in disease treatment by using fine needles to pierce *Jingmai*. Unfortunately, because this finding was so ancient, later medical experts did not comprehend its real meaning and many misinterpretations occurred.

"Those who do not understand the essence talk pointlessly and endlessly." This phrase refers to the above mentioned tendency towards misinterpretation. "For those who know the essence, one sentence is enough." That is to say, for those who know the real meaning of *Jie*, one sentence is enough. "The so-called *Jie* are places where *Shen Qi* travels in and out, they are neither skin, muscles, tendons nor bones" expresses the meaning of *Jie* in one pithy sentence.

By the time *Ling Shu* was published Chinese medical experts had developed the deepest and the most authoritative interpretation of *Jie* and "Crossings of *Jie*, 365 junctions." Here the author presented his conclusions based on his anatomical, physiological, and pathological studies, and then abstained from referring to other medical principles and issues.

However, after my in-depth study of the expert's summary of the special function of *Jie* and its scope, I found that the *Jie* is not a joint in the anatomical sense, nor is it the junction of joints. A joint in the anatomical sense cannot be the place where *Shen Qi* (spirit energy) travels in and out. Rather, it belongs to the category of bone structure. The true meaning of *Jie*, therefore, refers to the anterolateral and posterolateral spinal tracts and neurofilments, which are the pathways for the outgoing impulses of nerve motion and the incoming sensory information. They are not, as is sometimes believed, skin, muscles, tendons, and bones.

Based on this view we know that the phrase "Junctions where *Qi* flows and counter flows, exits and enters" refers to the somatic nerves that are formed by crossing spinal nerves. This term thus offers a simple and accurate expression of *Jingmai* in the human body, revealing the true meaning of the term "*Shen Qi* (spirit energy) travels in and out." Unfortunately, most medical experts have not understood its true meaning, and it is heartbreaking to see how their misconceptions have so negatively affected the inheritance and development of Chinese acupuncture.

4. The Three "*Qi*" ("its")

"*Qi*" is a pronoun meaning either "it, them, its" or "that, those." For the sake of brevity, this paragraph uses three "its" to refer to the body part that contains a disease.

For example "Use fine needles to open up its *Jingmai*" means to pierce the *Jingmai* associated with a disease using fine needles. "Regulate its *Qi* and blood" means to regulate the *Qi* and blood of the body part that contains the disease. "Managing its junction where *Qi* flows and counters flow, exits and enters" means to manage the *Jingmai* that control or are associated with the disease.

In light of this context, to apply acupuncture to the *Jingmai* does not mean that the doctor randomly pierces points over the entire body. Instead, acupuncturists must first identify the location of the disease and then pierce the specific *Jingmai* that control or are associated with the disease. By so doing they regulate the *Qi* and blood of the body part that contains the disease, enhance the function of the *Jingmai* associated with this disorder, and thus cure the disease. Unfortunately, previous interpretations failed to take into account the proper use of the term "its." As a result, the meaning of the text was distorted, making it difficult to understand, and even more difficult for future generations to apply.

5. "Passed it on to the future generations, it is necessary to make clear rules."
"Passed it on to the future generations, make legislation to protect it."

Here "it" means specifically to the use of "fine needles to open up its *Jingmai*, regulate its *Qi* and blood, manage its junction of flow and counter flow and entering/exiting points."

The conviction among ancient Chinese medical experts that *Jingmai* treatment can and should be passed on generationally ranks as an important prophesy in the history of medicine, demonstrating the wisdom and courage of the early doctors who championed it. All the more unfortunate then that so many flawed interpretations (such as the one above) have been made in the name of this great text – interpretations that deprive future generations of their promised legacy, and that promote the compromised system of acupuncture that is practiced so widely today.

*F*urthermore, we know that the sentences "Use fine needles to open up its *Jingmai*, regulate its *Qi* and blood, manage its junction of flow and counter flow and entering/exiting points" and "Passed it on to the future generations, make legislation to protect it" are highly specialized interpretations written in a kind of technical language of the time. If readers are not equipped with clinical knowledge of this language and not experienced in related research, they will never penetrate the meaning of the text in an accurate way. Indeed, in order to interpret these writings accurately it is necessary to understand the meaning of this technical language along with every detail of its special symbolism. Additionally, the text is written in a question and answer form, and each part is correlated (to every other part), making it a unified whole. For this reason, if interested parties are to interpret this writing correctly they need to read the entire text thoroughly and study the inter-relationships between each part – this, rather than simply reading random or isolated paragraphs.

(C) The special value and significance

This text has extraordinary value and great significance, for it accurately summarizes the method of using different types of needles to acupuncture different tissues in the body. This passage affirms the medical wisdom of using fine needles to pierce the most sensitive parts of the body i.e., the *Jingmai*. In clinical practice it advocates the use of subtle instruments such as (in today's world) fine filiform needles that gently pierce the *Jingmai* and generate immediate responses (the arrival of *Qi*), thus achieving effective healing. The text also explains the healing mechanism of acupuncture *Jingmai* for managing *Qi* and blood of the body parts that contain disease. The term "*shun ni chu ru zhi hui*" further explains the workings of the *Jingmai* and confirms the fact that using fine needles in acupuncture can make the *Jingmai* stronger. (Interestingly, the text compares the process of transformation of a patient receiving acupuncture to the emergence of a butterfly from a cacoon.) In the process it helps acupuncture make the leap into the modern world of scientific theory – just as it was foretold long ago.

From its origins *Ling Shu* was highly respected by doctors and generations of medical experts who developed it according to their own local perspectives. However, due to incorrect understanding and lack of seriousness acupuncture *Jingmai* was distorted in many ways. This is a great tragedy for Chinese acupuncture and has had catastrophic consequences on today's clinical practice (such as the use of fine needles to directly supplement *Qi* deficiency and drain *Qi* excess). Also in error is the theory that considers the *Jingmai* to be a unique system different and separate from the actual nerves and vessels of the nervous system. What creates such misapprehensions? Generally speaking, a partial and incomplete reading of the text. In order to address this problem and associated issues, we should use the given text to deal with related problems, a task that in the end should prove relatively easy. However, if we try to address the current situation and related problems with other methods, we will find these methods useless. This, in a nutshell, shows the relevance and great value of the ancient text we are dealing with.

In short, the text shines with the wisdom of the ancients and with their hope and firm belief in the healing power of the *Jingmai*. This work is a milestone, a fossil museum, and an exhibition hall rolled into one. Indeed, unless you read it attentively you will never truly understand Chinese acupuncture and the purpose/meaning of the *Ling Shu*. Motivated students should read this text often, strive to understand it correctly, and take it deeply to heart so that they can help restore its original teachings and make it better serve the goals of modern healing practice everywhere.

III. "A poor doctor only looks for the physical location of an acupoint, while a superior doctor seeks the spirit (*Shen*)." The spirit" mentioned here is wondrous; it is like a distinguished guest entering our door; without seeing the disease, how can one know the cause?"

Ling Shu - Nine Needles and Twelve Yuan-Source Points says: "A poor doctor only looks for the physical location of an acupoint, while a superior doctor seeks the spirit

(*Shen*) in the point. The spirit is wondrous; it is like a distinguished guest entering our door; without seeing the disease, how can one know the cause?"

Although this text is taken from the *Nine Needles and Twelve Source Points* it was written earlier than the *Ling Shu*. See Chapter 3 for a detailed interpretation.

I think the interpretation of the *Ling Shu*, Chapter 3 is largely incorrect. It completely contradicts the meaning of the original passage.

"A poor doctor only looks for the physical location of an acupoint, while a superior doctor seeks the spirit (*Shen*)" means that a poor doctor only knows how to apply needles to the acupuncture points, while a superior doctor knows how to acupuncture the *Jingmai* within these points – the somatic nerves.

"The spirit is wondrous; it is like a distinguised guest in the door" means that *Shen* is very mysterious; it is like an honored guest who resides within the points themselves. The *Shen* mentioned in this passage actually refers to *Jingmai*- the somatic nerves. "Without seeing the disease, how can one know the cause?" means that if a doctor does not observe and understand a particular disease he can never understand the origins of that disease.

T.N. Chan Interpretation: Based on observations made by Dr. Jiao, *it could be said that the ancient Chinese system of Jingmai is more or less equivalent to the modern concept of the human nervous system. As such, this system plays a central part in linking up the physical body to the Divine Matrix or Higher Intelligence – the Tao, if you will. Critical to this connection is the Shen mentioned above and throughout the following text. The Shen, which means "spirit" or "diety," is also one of the three fundamental life energies, along with Qi and Jing. Shen flows into us, out of us, through us, and around us, connecting us to the universe and representing, as it were, the divine plasma that we are all engulfed in, as well as the divine force that dwells within each living person. In other words, we are all made up of the same stardust materials that originated in an infinitesimally small space the size of a quark at the moment of the Big Bang.*

It can be said that just as we could connect to the Internet through WiFi to anywhere in the world, we could connect to the Divine Matrix through our Shen. "Where is the Internet?" one might be asked. "Where is this digital information we can access at any time with a simple username and password?" Answer: It is nowhere, yet it is everywhere. It is all around us, like the Spirit or Shen itself. This means, in turn, that when acupuncturists insert a needle into one of the Jingmai points, this needle serves to "download" cosmic healing Shen into a patient's body, much in the way that digital messages are downloaded by WiFi onto our personal computers. This "download" is made possible since the Jingmai interfaces the physical with the etheric. In other words, the Divine Matrix is not only outside of us in the cosmos, but inside of us in the very network of neurons that weaves its way throughout our bodies; it is the acupuncture needle that connects the two. As the Chinese sages have always maintained, "All things in the universe are interrelated."

Based on the content of this writing, it is estimated that it may have been written as long as 3,000 years ago. According to this notion, Chinese medical experts knew how to find the *Jingmai* within the acupuncture points – the somatic nerves – using fine needle acupuncture almost before the invention of written language.

IV. Analysis of "A poor doctor only knows how to look for the physical joints (*Guan*) while the superior doctor knows how to find the gate mechanism in the point (*Ji*)... This is the complete explanation of the *Tao* of acupuncture."

Ling Shu Chapter 1 - Nine Needles and Twelve Source Points says: "A poor doctor only knows how to look for the physical joints (*Guan*) while the superior doctor knows how to find the gate mechanism in the point (*Ji*). The movement of *Ji* never exceeds its space. When we observe it from the outside, *Ji* activity appears tranquil in the space it occupies. It appears to have only a slight movement. Its coming cannot be met and its going cannot be followed or grasped. Those who understand the gate mechanism are able to pierce the points precisely without missing a hair's breadth. Those who do not understand the gate mechanism will miss the timing of *Qi*. Piercing points in a random way is useless. Knowing where *Qi* is coming from and where it is going and timing of *Qi* to get the best result is important. This phenomenon is really wondrous. The poor doctor remains in the dark (about it), while the superior doctor knows all these (important facts). When *Qi* goes away, it is called 'counter flow'; when it arrives, it is called 'flow.' When counter flow and flow are grasped, positive actions can be practiced without question. If you meet (counter) *Qi* and deplete it, how can the excess not be drained? Follow and reinforce it, how can the deficiency not be filled? Countering and following the *Qi*, following the *Qi* dynamics with one's mind, this is the complete explanation of the *Tao* of acupuncture."

Although this scripture is from the *Ling Shu* its origin dates back to an earlier time. This fact is explained in detail in *Ling Shu Chapter 3 - Explanation of Small Needles*. Generations of doctors have tried to interpret this passage, but most never considered perspectives outside the framework of *Ling Shu Chapter 3 - Explanation of Small Needles*. When I checked the original scripture I found that the interpretation was patently incorrect. Indeed, some interpretations directly contradicted the original meaning of the passage. If the study of acupuncture follows these erroneous interpretations, the passage "A poor doctor only knows to look for the physical joints (*Guan*) while the superior doctor knows how to find the gate mechanism (*Ji*). This is the complete explanation of the *Tao* of acupuncture" would be burdened with mistakes and never be accurately revealed to the world. Therefore, only the interpretation based on the true meaning of the text can return the valuable information and scientific research embodied in this text to its rightful place in Chinese acupuncture theory.

The following are interpretations based on the original meaning of the text: "A poor doctor only knows to look for the physical joints (*Guan*) while the superior doctor knows how to find the gate mechanism in the point (*Ji*)" means that a poor doctor treats disease only by working with the physical acupuncture points, while a superior doctor knows how to treat diseases by acupuncturing the *Ji* within these points. "The movement of *Ji* never exceeds its space" means that *Ji* itself (inside the space) can move, but its movement never exceeds its space. This interpretation calls our attention to the fact that *Ji* is specified as an object (or tissue); it is definitely not *Qi*. The term "Kong" does not mean points because the movement of *Ji* does not exceed its space. "Its" refers to *Ji* itself. Thus "never exceeds its space" means that *Ji* does not leave its space (area). "When we observe it from the outside *Ji* activity appears tranquil in the space it occupies. It appears to have only a slight movement" means that *Ji* is in its space. It appears to be quiescent when observed from the outside, and its movement is very subtle (this conclusion is probably derived from anatomy and the direct examination of *Ji*).

"Its coming cannot be met and its going cannot be chased" means that in the space of *Ji* (inside the space) information can be transmitted in and out. This transmission is natural and wondrous – an observer could never observe its workings from the outside, a conclusion most likely derived from complicated physiological experiments. "Those who understand the gate mechanism are able to pierce the points precisely without missing a hair's breadth" means that those who understand the essence of *Ji* can pierce it without being off by a hair's breadth. "Those who do not understand the key point will miss the timing of *Ji*" means, metaphorically speaking, that those who do not understand the essence of *Ji* can – metaphorically speaking – pull the trigger but the gun will not shoot. In other words, if doctors do not understand the timing of *Ji*, and if they practice acupuncture only by randomly piercing the points they will never master their art. "Knowing where it is coming from, where it is going and the timing *Qi* to get the best results are all important" means that if doctors know the coming and going of *Qi* they will easily pierce *Ji*. "This phenomenon is really wondrous. The inferior doctor remains in the dark, while the superior doctor knows all these (important facts)" means that inferior doctors cannot understand the ways and means of acupuncture practice in a deep way; only superior doctors can plumb its subtle secrets.

"When *Qi* goes away, it is called counter flow; when it arrives, it is called flow. When counter flow and flow are grasped, positive (healing) actions can be taken without (doubts or) questions" means that the direction that is contrary to the "arrival of *Qi*" is the direction of counter flow, while the direction of the "arrival of *Qi*" is the direction of flow. Knowing the meaning of flow and counter flow, one can boldly practice acupuncture with no further questions. "(If you) meet (counter) *Qi* and deplete it, how can the excess not be drained? Follow and reinforce it, how can the deficiency not be filled?" means that if we counter the arrival of *Qi* and drain it, how can we avoid weakening the "arrival of *Qi*"? If we chase and push in, how can we not strengthen the "arrival of *Qi*"? "Countering and following the *Qi*, following the *Qi* dynamics with one's mind" means that by pushing in the needle and pulling it out we can adjust the intensity of the "arrival of *Qi*". "This is the complete explanation of the *Tao* of acupuncture" means that the above dictums are all basic to the correct practice of basic acupuncture.

According to the interpretation of the above passage, we know that as early as 3,000 years ago Chinese medical experts used the word "*Ji*" in the proper context and had a deep understanding of its meaning. Also, that the superior doctors knows how to treat disease by piercing the *Ji* within the points. When it comes to piercing with needles, the direction that can trigger the "arrival of *Qi*" is the correct direction, while the direction that weakens the "arrival of *Qi*" is the wrong direction. Finally, the methods of "Meet" and "Chase" can be used to adjust the intensity of the "arrival of *Qi*."

Medical experts in ancient China described *Ji* in a vivid and mysterious way. But what is *Ji*, really? According to studies and to knowledge of modern anatomy and physiology, it is clear that the somatic nerves are in many ways astonishingly similar to the *Ji* described by ancient Chinese medical experts. Therefore, we can assume that as early as 3,000 years ago Chinese medical practitioners had systematically summarized their technique of using fine needles to stimulate the somatic nerves. Even today such skill and wisdom ranks high in the annals of world medicine. At a time, when the level of medical practice throughout the world was still primitive and people knew very little about the structure of the human body, ancient Chinese doctors were intimately familiar with the workings of the somatic nerves, and were busy inventing scientific techniques to treat a host of human diseases.

The above facts fill me with awe and make me deeply appreciate the wisdom, passion, devotion and nobility of ancient Chinese medical experts. In essence, what they explored was a marvelous path of heaven. As early as 3,000 years ago they used Chinese needling techniques to lead them into the heaven realm of science. For this reason, we must understand their heritage correctly, and pass it on to coming generations with great sincerity.

Truth is the most important thing.

Comments on whether the medical art of Chinese needling is scientific should be based on facts. The analysis of the passage "A poor doctor only knows to look for the physical joints (*Guan*) while the superior doctor knows how to find *Ji* – the gate mechanism. This is the complete explanation of the *Tao* of acupuncture" has proved from one perspective that Chinese needling practice is indeed scientific.

V. Analysis of "For those who practice acupuncture, (treat) deficiency by filling, excess by draining, chronic stagnation by eliminating and over abundance of evil *Qi* by withdrawing."

Ling Shu Chapter 1 - Nine Needles and Twelve Source Points says: "For those who practice acupuncture, treat deficiency by filling, excess by draining, chronic stagnation by eliminating and over abundance of evil *Qi* by withdrawing." *Ling Shu Chapter 3 - Explanation of Small Needles* says: "Treat deficiency by filling." This phrase refers to using the fill method when there is deficiency at *Qi* kou. "(Treat) excess by draining" refers to using the draining method when there is excess at *Qi* kou. "Chronic stagnation by eliminating" means to eliminate the blood and tissues that have become corrupted. "Over abundance of evil *Qi* by withdrawing" tells us that if there is excessive activity in the *Jingmai* this means pathogenic factors are present. Su Wen Chapter 54 - Explanation of Needles says: "When the tip of the needle feels empty first and then solid this means there is heat under the needle, and that the solidness of *Qi* is caused by this heat" "Man ze xie zhi" means that when there is coldness under the needle a deficiency of *Qi* is present. "Chronic stagnation by eliminating" refers to letting out bad blood. "Abundance of evil *Qi* by withdrawing" means we do not press when pulling out the needle to let out the evil *Qi*. *Huang Di Nei Jing Ling Shu-Explained in Modern Chinese*[1] says: "The deficiency syndrome should be treated with the filling method so that the positive *Qi* can be supplemented. The full and excess syndrome should be treated with the draining method, so that the pathogenic factors of diseases can be eliminated. For symptoms caused by chronic stagnation of blood, the blood should be drained in order to eliminate the pathogenic factors that have stagnated in the body. For syndromes caused by the over-activity of pathogenic factors and pathogenic factors overcoming the positive factors, the draining method should be used to let out the pathogenic factors of disease, turning it from excess to emptiness."

Different contemporary interpretations of *Huang* Di Nei *Jian-Ling Shu* tend to be similar because most are based on *Ling Shu* - Explanation of Small Needles Chapter 3. In fact, these interpretations are generally incorrect and totally distort the meaning of the original passage. In my opinion, the original meaning was derived by Chinese doctors, and from the experience and thoughtful reflection that comes from treating patients with fine needles (including filiform needles). When performing acupuncture, all doctors should insert the required needles at certain points on the body and then attempt to pierce the *Jingmai*. If the tip of the needle feels empty when it is pushed in (or soft, with little resistance, or again, with no special feeling), this is proof that the needle has not yet reached the *Jingmai*. At this time, one should pierce further in or change the direction and pierce again till the *Jingmai* is reached. When there is a sudden increase of resistance at the tip of the needle or a feeling of firmness, this sensation reflects the exact meaning of "(treat) deficiency by filling".

"(Treat) excess by draining" means when *De Qi* is too full it should be drained a little. *De Qi* is a phenomenon that ordinarily occurs when *Jingmai* is pierced. Sometimes if *De Qi* is too strong and the patient cannot bear the sensation, the doctor should withdraw the needle a bit so that *De Qi* is reduced. Based on the sentence "(Treat) excess by draining," the technique of adjusting the intensity of *De Qi* was conceived. "Chronic stagnation by eliminating" refers to the special sensation that occurs when the tip of the

---

[1] *Huang Di Nei Jing-Ling Shu Explained in Modern Chinese* Edited by Wang Hong Tu, People's Medical Publishing House 2006 First Edition.

needle reaches (touches) the bones, tendons, or scar tissues and cannot penetrate any further. The appropriate action at this point is to withdraw the needle a little, change the direction, and then re-pierce the point. "Over abundance of evil *Qi* by withdrawing" refers to the severe shivering and numbness or pain that occurs when the needle pierces the *Jingmai*. Patients usually cannot bear this sensation, and many medical experts view it as a sign that pathogenic factors are present. When this sensation occurs the doctor should withdraw the needle a little. The pathogenic factors will then be relieved. This is the original meaning of the sentence "over abundance of evil *Qi* by withdrawing."

I think this interpretation not only matches the original meaning of the passage but clearly describes the core method of using fine needles to treat disease. Time flies like a weaver's shuttle and the world has experienced great changes. Even though 3,000 years have passed, these clinical techniques are still used on a regular basis by Chinese physicians. Thus, this passage not only has great scientific value but offers important medical advice that all modern practitioners would be wise to follow.

VI. New Understandings on "Slow then rapid is excess. Rapid then slow is deficiency."

Ling Shu Chapter 1 - Nine Needles and Twelve Source Points says: "'The Great Essentials' says: 'Slow then rapid is excess. Rapid then slow is deficiency.'" Based on this statement we know that this sentence is taken from *Ling Shu Chapter 1 - Nine Needles and Twelve Source Points*, and that its principles originated in a famous medical text called *The Great Essentials*. While there is no clear evidence of when *The Great Essentials* was written, many historical references, both ancient and modern, refer to it. Another important text Su Wen specifically mentions that *The Great Essentials* was, in fact, an ancient scripture. According to this reference, we can estimate that "Slow then rapid is excess. Rapid then slow is deficiency" embodies a very old concept and may well date from the ancient era.

Since the appearance of "Slow then rapid is excess. Rapid then slow is deficiency" in *The Great Essentials* medical experts have considered it to be of great importance. There are, however, different interpretations regarding its exact meaning, and it has influenced acupuncture technique in a number of different ways. Among them, *Ling Shu Chapter 3 - Explanation of Small Needles* says: "'Slow then rapid is excess' means insert the needle slowly and withdraw it rapidly. 'Rapid then slow is deficiency' means rapidly insert the needle and slowly withdraw it." This interpretation was then quoted relatively often, resulting in yet more deviations. It finally evolved into the "rapid and slow tonify and drain" method. This special method of "tonify the deficiency, drain the excess" was then passed down to the present day.

Among older medical texts there are different interpretations. For example, the text Su Wen Chapter 54 - Explanation of Needles says: "Slow then rapid is excess" which means withdraw the needle slowly and press it rapidly. Likewise, "Rapid then slow is deficiency" tells us to withdraw the needle rapidly and press it slowly.

In my view, both of these interpretations are incorrect. Why? Because the sentences "Slow then rapid is excess. Rapid then slow is deficiency" do not actually describe how a doctor, while inserting and withdrawing needles, fills the deficiency and drains the excess through slow and rapid movement. Rather, it describes the particular experience of piercing points on certain parts of the body. Thus, according to the speed and intensity of resistance that suddenly occurs at the tip of the needle, one can tell if the *Jingmai* have been pierced or not. The mechanics of this method require the doctor to pierce the skin, then attempt to find and pierce the *Jingmai*. When the tip of the needle is about to reach the depth of *Jingmai*, the doctor gently pushs the needle in or gently twists it in. If a tightening feeling is felt at the tip of the needle, and if a sudden increase of resistance results, this means that the tip of the needle has successfully pierced the *Jingmai*, a sensation that is often referred to as "firm." When a doctor pushes the needle in or twists it in, and the feeling at the tip of the needle is soft or if there is little resistance despite the fact that the piercing speed is fast and hard, this means that the needle is still in the emptiness (that is, it has not yet pierced *Jingmai*), a condition that is referred to as "empty." Although thousands of years have passed, these sentences still offer the best advice for piercing the *Jingmai* and treating disease.

The Great Essentials describes the practice of piercing *Jingmai*. Through comparative studies of neuron-anatomy and knowledge of physiology and needling tests, it has been found that this practice is the same as that of piercing the somatic nerves.

According to this statement, we know that at a very ancient time Chinese medical experts began to use fine needles for treating disease, and that by so doing they accumulated valuable experience concerning whether or not to pierce the *Jingmai*.

VII. Analysis of "Pierce and *Qi* does not arrive, do not ask how many times; pierce and *Qi* arrives, remove the needle and no more piercing."

In *Ling Shu Chapter 1 - Nine Needles and Twelve Source Points* it says: "(If you) pierce and *Qi* does not arrive, do not ask how many times; pierce and *Qi* arrives, remove the needle and perform no more piercing" This means: (If you attempt to) pierce (the point) and *Qi* does not arrive, do not ask how many times (how many attempts you have made); (but if you) pierce the point and *Qi* arrives, remove the needle and perform no more piercings. The earliest interpretation on record of this scripture is in the *Huang Di Nei Jing Ling Shu* - Notes and Elaborative Explanations by Mr. Ma Shi, composed in the *Ming* Dynasty. He wrote: "If *Qi* does not arrive after piercing, one should not ask (how many) times but anticipate. It is like waiting for an honorable guest and not knowing that it is already sunset. If one pierces (the point) and *Qi* arrives immediately, remove the needle." The interpretations of future medical experts are mostly based on this passage.

I think this interpretation does not match the original meaning of the scripture. The phrase "Pierce and *Qi* does not arrive, do not ask how many times," specifically refers to "pierce." The text does not mention the terms "anticipate" or "wait." Mr. Ma Shi added the phrases "to anticipate" and also "it is like waiting for an honorable guest, one does not know it is already sunset." These latter additions are in my opinion superfluous and unnecessary. By including them the author not only failed to explain the text clearly but has violated its original meaning.

The fact is that between 2,500 and 3,000 years ago Chinese medical experts confirmed that if *Qi Zhi* (the "arrival of *Qi*") occurs when performing acupuncture with fine needles, healing effects will assuredly follow. Therefore, a number of efforts have been made to study this practice. Different techniques to trigger *Qi Zhi* have appeared over the years including those that focus on the number of times a piercing takes place (three times, six times, nine times, etc.), and those that focus on the depth that the needle reaches when piercing (shallow, medium, deep, etc.). Over the centuries, applying in-depth study and careful analysis, medical experts who were experienced in clinical practice finally concluded that "Pierce and *Qi* does not arrive, do not ask how many times; pierce and *Qi* arrives, remove the needle and do no more piercing" summarizes all the techniques that trigger *Qi Zhi*. Although this conclusion is based on experience, it is also clear that *Qi Zhi* is triggered by needling, not by waiting.

When discussing the technique of using fine needles to treat disease, *Ling Shu Chapter 1 - Nine Needles and Twelve Yuan-Source Points* features this passage at the end. Today it is regarded as the sole standard that doctors should use when deciding whether or not to pierce *Jingmai*, and as such it represents the very core technique of needling *Jingmai*. Clinical practitioners cannot literally see the *Jingmai*, moreover; they can only estimate the location and depth of the nerves while piercing. If they miss the nerves on the first try, they should change the direction and depth, then pierce again till *Qi* arrives (which means that *Jingmai* is successfully pierced). Therefore, we can affirm the saying that "the arrival of *Qi* is the proof that *Jingmai* is pierced".

Due to different understandings of the text, different techniques have evolved over the centuries. After 2,500 years of this development the core technique of needling *Jingmai* (the phrase "Pierce and *Qi* does not arrive, do not ask how many times; pierce and *Qi* arrives, remove the needle and no more piercing.") has become one of many needling techniques. This evolution not only removed the technique from its core status, but made the *Jingmai* (somatic nerves) mysterious and incomprehensible.

Fortunately, clinical practitioners have always favored and preferred using this technique. Today it is not only in common use but is the best way to achieve assured healing effects in clinical practice.

If the status of this technique can be restored it will improve the healing effects in clinical practice and will benefit the discussion of needling *Jingmai* (somatic nerves) to treat disease.

VIII. Analysis of "The essence of needling is that once *Qi* arrives an effect is generated. This effect appears quickly, as when the wind is blowing away the clouds and the sky suddenly turns clear and blue. This process describes the complete *Tao* of needling."

Ling Shu Chapter 1 - Nine Needles and Twelve Source Points says: "The essence of needling is that once *Qi* arrives an effect is generated. This effect appears quickly, as if the wind is blowing away the clouds and the sky suddenly turns clear and blue. This process describes the complete *Tao* of needling."

"The essence of needling is that once *Qi* arrives an effect is generated" means that the most essential point to note about needling is that once the "arrival of *Qi*" occurs healing effects are assured. "This effect appears so quickly as when the wind blows away the clouds, the sky suddenly turns clear and blue" means that this healing effect is totally predictable, coming as quickly (and surely) as when the wind blows away the clouds and the sky suddenly becomes clear and blue. "This process describes the complete *Tao* of needling" means this is the basic principle of needling to treat disease, and that nothing else need be says (on the subject).

The text was originally written as a summary of needling practice. It describes in an affirmative way the best needling techniques for bringing about unique healing effects. The implied meaning is that this technique brings speedy and good healing, and that other methods pale in comparison.

Various understandings of the text evolved into different techniques of needling. After more than 2,000 years of this evolution the technique of needling *Jingmai* to trigger the "arrival of *Qi*" and achieve unique healing effects is still only one of many different needling procedures. This loss of the true understanding of *Jingmai* has reduced the healing effect of acupuncture, and has contributed to a severe deterioration in its clinical practice.

IX. Tentative Analysis of "Crossings of *Jie*, 365 junctions. For those who know the essence, one sentence is enough, while those who do not know talk pointlessly and endlessly. The so-called *Jie* are places where *Shen Qi* travels in and out; they are neither skin, muscles, tendons nor bones."

Ling Shu Chapter1 - Nine Needles and Twelve Yuan-Source Points says: "Crossings of *Jie*, 365 junctions. For those who know the essence, one sentence is enough, while those who not know talk pointlessly and endlessly. The so-called *Jie* are places where *Shen Qi* travels in and out; they are neither skin, muscles, tendons nor bones."[2] After this text was published medical practitioners used and interpreted it in many varying ways. Different interpretations of *Huang* Di Nei *Jing* mostly interpreted the *Jie* as "the gap in the articular cavity" or in "the physical joints." In my view, both these notions are incorrect. First, the text insists that, "they are not skin, muscles, tendons and bones." It also clearly

---

[2] *Explanations of Huang Di Nei Jing-Ling Shu*, edited and written by Department of Chinese Medicine, Nanjing University of Traditional Chinese Medicine, Shanghai Science and Technology Publishing House, July, 1997, fifth edition.

points out that the *Jie* are not bones but something different. The physical joints and the articular cavities belong to the bone category, not to the skin, and because of this misunderstanding many interpretations are misleading and unconvincing. Second, it is incorrect to say that all of the 365 acupuncture points on the body are located in the gap of the articlular cavities. Many of these points (for example, Cheng Shan, Cheng Jing, Zu San Li, Nei *Guan*, and Wai *Guan*) are not in the gap of the articular cavities at all. Third, it is important to understand that the gap of the articular cavities is actually the place where *Shen Qi* (spirit energy) travels in and out. Moreover, there is mainly joint fluid in the joints, and it is an obvious impossibility that these fluids form junctions that allow the *Shen Qi* to travel in and out.

In order to interpret this text, we need to understand the basic meaning of *Jie* as well as its specific definition.

This text can be divided into three parts. The first part tells us that "crossings of *Jie*, 365 junctions" (there are 365 crossings of *Jie*, or junctions). It is very difficult to understand that this is the core of the argument. The following two parts serve only to illustrate this first. The second part tells us that "For those who know the essence, one sentence is enough; those who do not know talk pointlessly and endlessly." This statement means that "crossings of *Jie*, 365 junctions" are extremely difficult to understand. Those who understand its essence will be able to explain it in one sentence. Those who do not will talk endlessly (but never reach the truth in the matter). The third part tells us that "The so-called *Jie* are places where *Shen Qi* travels in and out; they are neither skin, muscles, tendons nor bones." Translated, this sentence clearly explains that *Jie* are not muscles, skin, tendons and bones, and that they allow *Shen Qi* to travel in and out. What variety of tissue in the human body comprises this special tissue of *Jie*? Where is it located? No one is certain. In order to find the *Jie* as described in the text, we must turn to anatomy and physiology, and make comparative studies of the tissues that are similar to *Jie* in terms of structure and function.

If such tissues can be found, we will then have proof that this text is entirely accurate, and thus we can verify its scientific value. I myself have found (in my own practice) that the anterolateral and posterolateral spinal tracts and neurofilments are, in fact, the *Jie* described in the text. Moreover, I have observed that the front and rear nerve roots (threads) join in sections, forming the front and rear roots. These two structures join and give shape of the spinal nerves which are similar to "Crossings of *Jie*" described in the text. Some of the spinal nerves pass through the foramen intervertebrales and then join together to form nerve plexus. They also converge and form different nerves that extend to the parts of the body that control various organs and tissues. Most of the nerves in the human body are capable of transmiting essential information (motion and sensory impulses) in and out, even though, as the text proclaims, they are not part of the skin, muscle, tendon and bone structures.

Long ago the famous Western physician Galen (130-200 AD) dissected a sheep and observed the structure of its brain. By so doing he discovered that there are empty "rooms" in the brain and "rooms" filled with fluids. This observation caused him to conclude that all sensations are recorded by the brain, and that all motions are triggered by this essential organ. Both, he believed, are caused by "fluids" flowing in and out of the brain. Galen's theory lasted for almost 1,500 years.

In 1751 a book titled The Experiment and Observation of Electricity proposed the theory that the human nervous system operates much like a network of "electrical cables" carrying electrical impulses to and fro throughout the body. Fifty years after publication of this book the Italian scientist Luigi Calvani and the German biologist Emil du Bois-Regmend proved that when electric impulses are sent through various nerves they stimulate tremors in the muscles. It was also discovered that the brain itself is capable of generating electrical impulses. These findings replaced Galen's theory that nerves connect to the brain via the in-flow and out-flow of fluids.

T. N. Chan Interpretation: Although some argue that when Galen spoke of "fluids," he actually refered to what we know to be Qi or energy flow.

Around 1810, the Scotsman Charles Bell observed that when he cut the back nerve roots (rear roots) and the abdominal nerve roots (front roots) of an experimental animal its muscles were paralyzed only if the nerve roots (front roots) in the abdomen were cut. In France, Francois Magendie then proved that the back nerve roots (rear roots) send sensory information into the spinal cord. Based on these discoveries, Bell and Magendie reasoned that the human nervous system is indeed similar to a set of electrical cables, but that some of these cables send information into the spinal cord and brain, and some send information out to the muscles. They observed that the anterior spinal roots contain only motor fibers, and that the posterior roots have only sensory fibers. They also proved that for each sensory nerve and motion nerve, the transmission of information runs exclusively one way. Finally, they showed that for most of their length the two types of nerves are wrapped together, separating only when they enter or leave the spinal cord.[3]

T. N. Chan Interpretation: The above historical facts show clearly that as early as the 18th century Western doctors knew that the front and rear nerve roots of the spinal cord and surrounding nerves transmit motional and sensory information. Today most books and atlases in neuron-anatomy published in the 20th century include detailed descriptions of the anterolateral and posterolateral spinal tracts and neurofilments.

The above information demonstrates that several centuries ago Western doctors understood the root system of the spinal cord, as well as the fact that the peripheral

---

[3] NEUROSCIENCE: *Exploring the Brain* by Mark F.Bear, Barry W.Connors, and Michael A.Paradiso. Translated by Wang Jian Jun, Higher Education Press, July, 2004, fifth edition.

nervous system has pathways that transmit motor and sensory information. In recent times, of couse, a great deal more scientific knowledge has been gained concerning the tracings in the anterolateral sulcus of spinal cord nerve roots (small) and posterior lateral sulcus of the nerve root (small).

All well and good. But it should also be pointed out that as early as 1,800 years ago medical experts in China, using anatomical and neuro-physical studies along with clinical observation, had already proved the existence of the sulcus of the spinal cord nerve roots (small) and the posterior lateral sulcus of the nerve root (thin) filament. They named these parts "Festival," theorizing that information is passed through the nerve roots (thin) fiber of the body from organ to organ. Early Chinese medical experts also observed the workings of the anterolateral and posterolateral spinal tracts and neurofilments, calling what they saw *Jie*. By so doing they confirmed that the somatic nerves transmit nerve information freely in and out along the anterolateral and posterolateral spinal tracts and neurofilments.

The "crossing of *Jie*" refer to the anterolateral and posterolateral spinal tracts and to the neurofilments. These tracts join together to form the front roots and the rear roots, ultimately combining to form the spinal nerves. After moving through multiple joints they turn into nerves in different parts of the body. The 365 acupuncture points that can be pierced are relatively fixed points on the somatic nerves. Therefore, ancient Chinese medical experts called them "Crossings of *Jie*, 365 hui."

To sum up, the statement that "*Jie* are places where *Shen Qi* travels in and out; they are neither skin, muscles, tendons nor bones" presents a conclusive summary of Chinese medical experts' researches in neuron anatomy and physiology. These achievements are extraordinary and continue to have great value (for Chinese medicine). We must attach great importance to them, pass them on seriously (to future generations), and study them deeply in order to confront human disease in a fully scientific way.

X. Reflections on "Observe the eyes; one can know (much from) their dilation and recovery."

Ling Shu Chapter 1 - Nine Needles and Twelve Source Points says: "Observe the eyes; one can know much from their dilation and recovery. *Ling Shu Chapter 3 - Explanation of Small Needles* interpreted this statement as meaning "The superior doctor knows how to observe the condition of the five organs by looking at the eyes. By knowing their size, examining whether they are slow moving or quick, smooth or astringent, one can tell where diseases are located." *Huang Di Nei Jing-Ling Shu Notes and Elaborative Explanations* (by Mr. Ma Shi, *Ming* dynasty) interpreted this statement as saying: "The situations of the five organs are revealed in the eyes. Therefore, if a superior doctor wants to know the patient's health status he will examine the eyes and will then know the disbursement and recovery of the positive *Qi*." *Future generations often interpreted his words as meaning "examining the gaze (or look) in the eyes of a patient." In my opinion, this interpretation does not accord with the original meaning of the text. In my opinion, "Observe the eyes, one can know much from their dilation and recovery" means that by examining the eyes one will know the disbursement and recovery of the eye pupils. In this context, *San* means loosened, dispersed from aggregation, while *Fu* means recovery, replication, and repetition. (*The New Dictionary*, *Ji*ling University Press, 2001, latest edition).

Modern medicine informs us that the pupils of our eyes are approximately the same size, that they are round and about ±0.3 cm in diameter. They are very sensitive to light, meaning that they shrink and dilate when stimulated by light of different intensities. In clinical examinations around the world it has always been known that when the pupils are simulated by relatively strong light they shrink, and that when the light source is removed they quickly recover their original size. The universal knowledge of these facts indicates that this method of diagnosing disease is not a modern invention, nor was it first used in the Western countries. Indeed, it was routinely used by ancient Chinese medical experts as long as 3,000 years ago. Unfortunately, due to incorrect interpretations through the centuries, it ended up buried and neglected in the text of the *Ling Shu - Nine Needles and Twelve Yuan-Source Points*, Chapter 1.

In modern medicine, the shape and size of the eye pupils and their response to light are used for diagnosing disease and injury. For example, if both pupils are dilated and their response to light ceases entirely, a patient is presumed to be clinically dead. In case of brain injury cranial pressure increases due to the formation of intracranial hematoma, especially epidural hematoma. In this situation, when the oculomotor nerves on the side of the injury are stimulated, the pupil on that side of the head shrinks. As the intracranial hematoma grows in size the oculomotor nerves are further pressed, leading to pupil dilation, decreased sensitivity to light, and in the worst case scenario total lack of response to light. If a clear diagnosis can be made during this period, and if the intracranial hematoma can be removed, the pressure to the oculomotor nerves is relieved and the size of the pupil and its response to light returns to normal.

If we can correctly understand and seriously utilize the statement "Observe the eyes, one can know much from their dilation and recovery," then we can significantly enhance the level of clinical diagnosis.

生顺发出

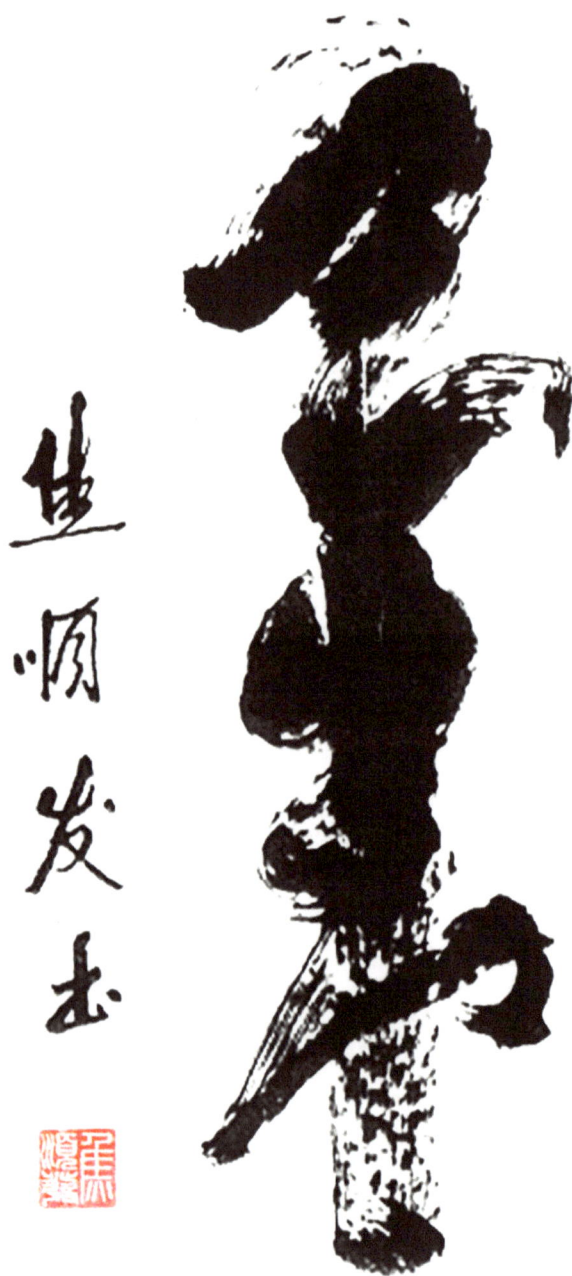

"*Qi*"
Calligraphy by Dr. Jiao

CHAPTER TWO

On Jingmai

———————

"The discovery of Du mai represents a major leap forward for the understanding of Jingmai in the human body. It not only presents Jingmai as a complete system; it also provides doctors with the power to determine life and death, to regulate (energy flow), and to balance (human energies). The discovery of Du mai also contributed to passages in Ling Shu - Nine Needles and Twelve Yuan-Source Points such as: "Using fine needles to open up its Jingmai, regulate its blood and Qi, and manage its junctions of flow and counter flow, and entering and exiting points." In short, the discovery of Du mai made great contributions to the art of fine needle acupuncture."

*M*edical experts in China began to study *Jingmai* in the human body as early as 4,000 years ago. Over the years they made great advancements in scientific research through extensive, deep and persistent research.

Ling Shu Chapter 1 - Nine Needles and Twelve Source Points has made great contributions to the study of *Jingmai*. It not only correctly expresses and illustrates human *Jingmai*, it passes down an understanding of them from experience based on reflections, research, and scientific discussion. The following is a discussion on some of the important content in this passage.

Section 2.1 - *Jingmai* in the Spinal Cord

By means of an in-depth study of spinal cord *Jingmai* ancient Chinese medical scholars confirmed that they are an important part of the entire *Jingmai* system. The author of the *Ling Shu* believed that the *Jie* discussed in the text is actually the junction of somatic *Jingmai* and spinal *Jingmai*, similar in structure to the entrance and exit of somatic *Jingmai* at the spinal *Jingmai*. (*Ji Li* means inside the spinal cord.) Chinese medical experts discovered long ago that an important part of *Jingmai* is located inside the spinal cord. They called this area "spinal *Jingmai*" for short.

I. The Spine

As we know, the bones in the spine are among the most important structural elements in the human body. As early as two thousand years ago, they were identified and catalogued by Chinese medical experts, and over the centuries they have been studied extensively in many parts of China. For example, the *Ling Shu Chapter 14 - Gu Du (On the Measurement of Bones)*, informs us that: "There are two and half *Cun* between the hair line on the back of neck and the back bone; between the first thoracic vertebra process and the coccygeal vertebrae there are 21 spinal bones three Chi long. The upper part is 1.41 *Cun*[4], *Qi* fen is below, and thus the first seven spinal bones up to the first thoracic vertebra process are 9.87 *Cun* in length. This is the measurement of normal human bones. It is used to measure the length of *Jingmai*."

---

[4] One *Cun* is about 1.5 cm.

II. Hollow in the spine

Ancient Chinese medical experts have long known and studied the hollows in the middle of the spine, referring to them at times as "rooms." For example, the *Su Wen-Gu Kong Lun* (*On the Hollows of Bones*), Chapter 60, tells us that: "The top space of the spine is above *Feng Fu*, the bottom space of the spine is at the coccygeal vertebrae. The space inside the spine is between the two hollows."

III. Jingmai in the hollow inside the spine

Medical experts in China conducted in-depth research while studying the hollows inside the spine thousands of years ago, and in the process achieved profound and fruitful results. The results of this research are summarized below:

(A) *The "Sui" of Jingmais*

Ancient Chinese medical experts called the marrow in the hollow of the spine "*Sui.*" The text *Su Wen-Gu Kong Lun*, Chapter 60 says: "The hollow of *Sui* is located three Fen behind the brain, below the sharp bone at the rim of the skull. One of them is at the upper space of the spine above *Feng Fu*." This passage likewise tells us that "The upper hollow of the spine above *Feng Fu*" is the space of *Sui*." Also, that within this hollow is *Sui.*" The text *Ling Shu*-Hai Lun (*On the Sea*), Chapter 33 informs us that "There is a sea of *Sui* in the human" and "The brain is the sea of *Sui*." This passage that informs us that *Sui* in the spaces of the spine is connected to the brain, which in turn is the sea of "*Sui.*"

(B) *The "Sea" of Jingmai*

Chinese medical experts long ago described the hollows in the spine as being like *the "sea" of Jingmai*. Examples of this metaphor are found in the text *Ling Shu-Five Sounds and Five Tastes*, Chapter 65, which says: "*Chong mai* and *Ren mai* both start from the embryo; they go upward inside the back (backbone), which is the sea of *Jing Luo* (*Jingmai*)." The text *Zhen Jiu Jia Yi Jing - Qi Jing Ba Mai* or *A-B Classic of Acupuncture and Moxibustion*, Chapter 2 tells us that: "*Chong mai* and *Ren mai* both start from the embryo, then go upward inside the back (inside the backbone) which is the sea of *Jing Luo* (*Jingmai*)." When we read these passages we should pay special attention to the word "sea," which is described as the junction point where all the "rivers and streams" of the body converge. Only when we deeply comprehend the meaning of this symbol can we understand what is meant when the ancients said that *Jingmai* all over the human body converge into a central "sea."

(C) *The Governor of Jingmai*

Medical experts in ancient China discovered (and identified) the governor of *Jing-mai* centuries ago. The word "*Du*" is a verb meaning to supervise, govern, monitor. Therefore, *Du mai* is the governor that supervises the other *Jingmai*. Many discussions about *Du mai* were collected in the text *Su Wen-Gu Kong Lun*, Chapter 60. *Nan Jing* conducted in-depth anatomical research on *Du mai* and found that it was located in the hollows inside the spinal column. The text *Nan Jing-Twenty-Eighth Nan* tells us: "*Du mai* starts from *Shu* point at the bottom of the spine, merges into the spinal column, goes upward to *Feng Fu*, and enters into the brain." (See Figure 2-4). In *Zhen Jiu Jia Yi Jing - Qi Jing Ba Mai*, Chapter 2 we read: "*Du mai* starts from the *Shu* point at the bottom of the spine, merges into the spinal column, goes upward to *Feng Fu*, and enters into the brain, its upper end goes to the nasal column, it is the sea of Yang mai." This passage not only borrowed the idea from *Nan Jing-Twenty-Eighth Nan* that *Du mai* is located in the space inside the spinal column; it also considered *Du mai* to be the sea of Yang mai.

The discovery of *Du mai* represents a major leap forward for the understanding of *Jingmai* in the human body. It not only presents *Jingmai* as a complete system; it also provides doctors with the power to determine life and death, to regulate (energy flow), and to balance (human energies). The discovery of *Du mai* also contributed to passages in *Ling Shu - Nine Needles and Twelve Yuan-Source Points* such as: "Using fine needles to open up its *Jingmai*, regulate its blood and *Qi*, and manage its junctions of flow and counter flow, and entering and exiting points." In short, the discovery of *Du mai* made great contributions to the art of fine needle acupuncture.

(D) The Pivot of Jingmai

Around 2,000 years ago Chinese medical scientists discovered that there are pivots of *Jingmais* throughout the human body. The *Xuan Shu* point in *Zhen Jiu Jia Yi Jing* is the name of a point. It is located at the lower border of the thirteenth vertebra (the first lumbar vertebra). Precisely speaking, *Xuan Shu* is located below the lower border of the thirteenth vertebra. This discovery helps us better understand the *Jingmai* located inside the hollow of the spinal column.

Generally speaking, as early as 2000 years ago medical scientists in ancient China had great success conducting in-depth research on the *Jingmai* inside the spinal column. According to ancient medical practitioners *Sui*, Hai, *Du*, *Shu* are all inside the hollw of the spine, and each has a special meaning. For example, *Sui* (marrow) describes the change of substance of *Jingmai* after *Jingmai* from all over the body enter the hollows of the spinal column. Hai (sea) describes how the *Jingmai* all over the body converge like numerous rivers on the hollow of the spinal column. *Du* (governor) describes how *Jingmai* all over the body converge into the hollow of spinal column, and how it governs the *Jingmai* throughout the entire body. *Shu* (pivot) refers to the marrow located on the lower border of the thirteenth vertebra inside the spinal column, and how it acts as a pivot for *Jingmai* all over the body. The above descriptions are clear and accurate. Unfortunately, over the centuries mistakes of interpretation have been made, causing the *Jingmai* inside the spinal column to become misunderstood by researchers.

IV. *Jie* of *Jingmai* inside the spinal column

"*Jie*"of *Jingmai* inside the spinal column is a new term, and this is the first time I have referred to it. Medical experts in ancient China discovered the *Jie* of *Jingmai* inside the spinal column centuries ago, and the information concerning it is very ancient. For example, in the ancient text *Zhen Jiu Jia Yi Jing-Zhen Dao*," Chapter 4, it says: "Crossings of *Jie*, 365 junctions. For those who know the essence, one sentence is enough; those who do not know talk pointlessly and endlessly. The so-called *Jie* are places where *Shen Qi* travels in and out; they are neither skin, muscles, tendons nor bones." *Ling Shu Chapter 1 - Nine Needles and Twelve Source Points* made a great contribution to Chinese medicine by using this passage to summarize the somatic *Jingmai* and to discuss the location and special functions of *Jie*. After I read it I could see that the *Jie* described in this text is not located inside the physical joints or articular cavities. Instead, they are on both sides of the *Du mai* in the space of the spinal column. These *Jie* allow *Shen Qi* (spirit energy) to travel in and out, and as stated previously, they are not composed of skin, muscles, tendons or bones. Based on this concept, the *Jie* described by ancient Chinese medical experts is located inside the space of the spinal column. I refer to it as "*Jie* of *Jingmai* inside the spinal column."

There are many books that characterize *Jingmai* in such terms as *Jingmai*, *Jiu Juan*, *Zhen Jing* and similar words and phrases. Why then did *Ling Shu Chapter 1 - Nine Needles and Twelve Source Points* chose this particular passage? I think it was done deliberately. It is likely that the author of this work decided to use this passage after he verified the location and functions of *Jingmai* through anatomic and physiological experiments. Unfortunately, the generations that followed did not understand the original text, and they failed to correctly interpret the intent and objectives of its authors. They mistakenly located the *Jie* of *Jingmai* at the physical joints and articular cavities. Thus, the original meaning of *Jie* of *Jingmai* in the text of *Ling Shu Chapter 1 - Nine Needles and Twelve Source Points* fell into obscurity. This was, of course, a huge error. Because of it, the somatic *Jingmai* in the human body is not (understood to be) merged into the "sea," and the *Du mai* remains isolated and is not considered to be the "governor" of *Jingmai*. Up to this day these misinterpretations seriously hinder the application, research, and development of *Jingmai* theory.

Are the descriptions of ancient medical experts correct? Are my analysis and interpretations right? It is not helpful to make empty assertions. We can only rely on facts.

Our physical bodies today have the same structure and function they did in ancient times. Therefore, we need only compare the structure and function of our body's workings with descriptions that have come down to us from medical experts in the past to ascertain their accuracy.

Over the past 2,000 years medical science has developed in many significant ways. Today physicians are not only well versed in the anatomy and physiological functions of the human body; they are familiar with its micro-structures and complex functions, and can attain information on physiological matters simply by consulting modern medical texts. The materials inside the spinal column and the hollows in the column are located deep within the body; they can only be seen by direct anatomical observation. If we open a book on human anatomy we will find that the spinal column of the human skeleton supports the torso and the head (see Figure 2-1).

Vertebral Column

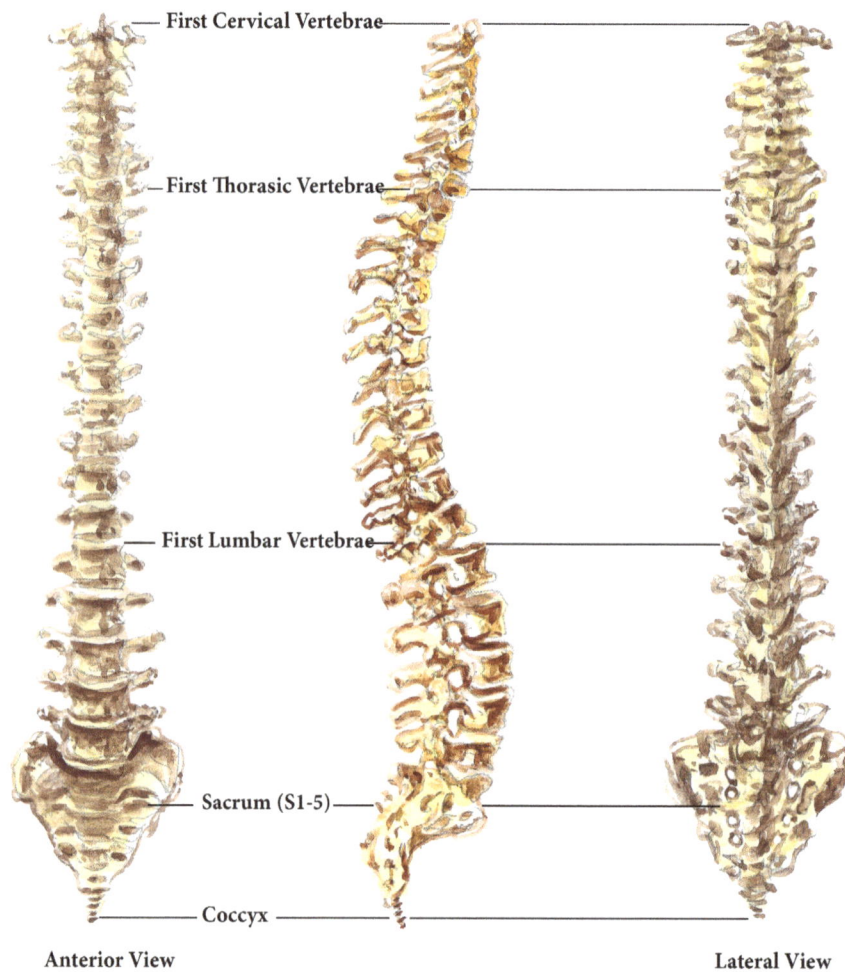

First Cervical Vertebrae

First Thorasic Vertebrae

First Lumbar Vertebrae

Sacrum (S1-5)

Coccyx

Anterior View   **Lateral View**

The human spinal column is described (in many texts) by ancient Chinese doctors (see Figure 2-2). Both the spinal column and the spinal ridge are part of the spine, and both have the same number of vertebrae. For example, there are seven cervical vertebrae on both, twelve thoracic vertebrae, five lumbar vertebrae, four sacral vertebrae and one coccygeal vertebra (see Figure 2-2).

Regional Characteristics of Vertebrae

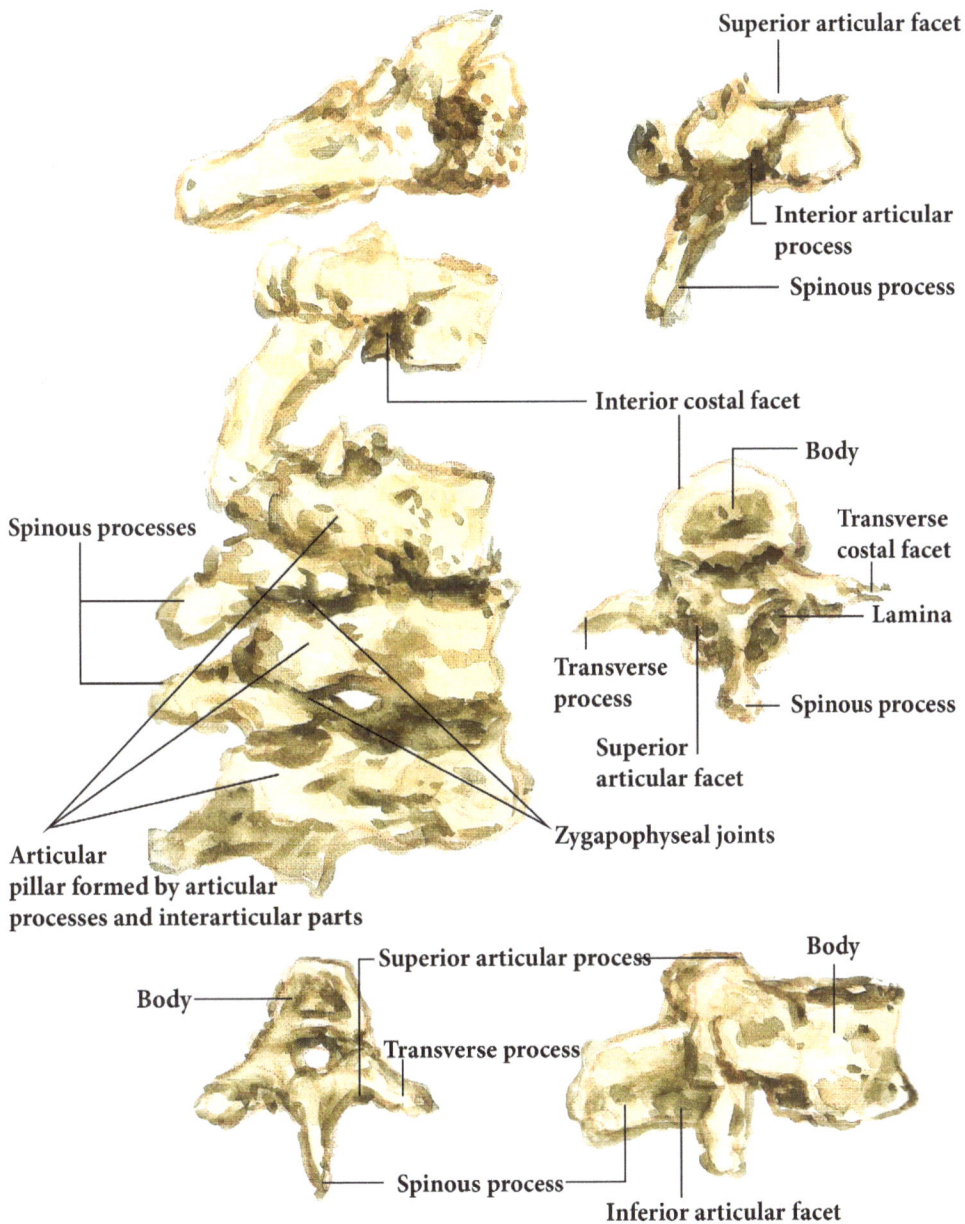

Superior articular facet

Interior articular process

Spinous process

Interior costal facet

Body

Transverse costal facet

Lamina

Spinous process

Transverse process

Superior articular facet

Zygapophyseal joints

Spinous processes

Articular pillar formed by articular processes and interarticular parts

Body

Superior articular process

Body

Transverse process

Spinous process

Inferior articular facet

[2-2]

The medical text *Ling Shu Chapter 14 - Gu Du* (*On the Measurement of Bones*) tells us that: "…of the top seven vertebrae, and between the first thoracic vertebra process, and in the coccygeal vertebra there are twenty one vertebrae." Also, that "The top seven vertebras" in the text are the same as the seven cervical vertebrae. These observations prove that medical scientists in ancient China counted the first seven vertebras based on vertebral segments and thoracic vertebrae, and that the segments below were counted by the spinous process. These facts confirm that the spinal bone spoken of in ancient Chinese medical texts is the spinal column (spinal vertebrae) described in modern medicine today.

Medical scientists in ancient China, as we have seen, discovered the hollows inside the spinal column. These hollows are analogous to the spinal apertures and vertebral canal studied in modern anatomy today. Both refer to the large spaces in the middle of the spine, as shown in Figure (2-3).

Bones of The Pelvis Anatomy

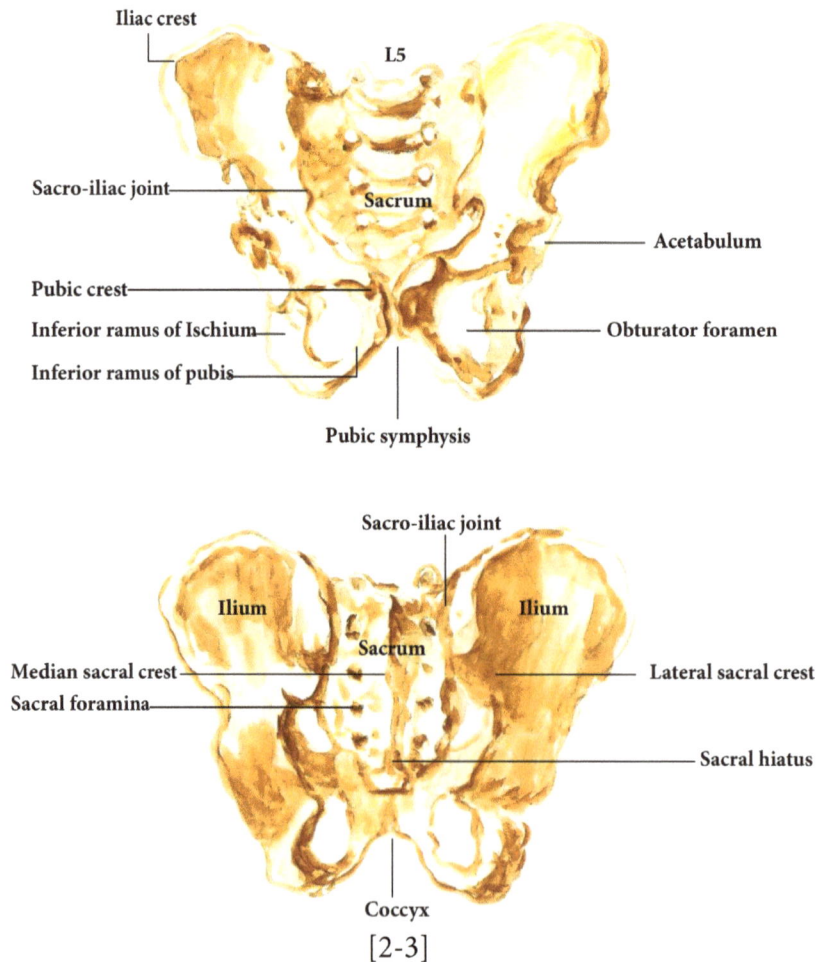

Iliac crest

L5

Sacro-iliac joint

Sacrum

Acetabulum

Pubic crest

Inferior ramus of Ischium

Obturator foramen

Inferior ramus of pubis

Pubic symphysis

Sacro-iliac joint

Ilium

Ilium

Sacrum

Median sacral crest

Lateral sacral crest

Sacral foramina

Sacral hiatus

Coccyx

[2-3]

According to this statement, the space inside the spinal column discovered by medical scientists in ancient China is the "vertebral canal" also described in modern medicine.

If we remove the spinous process and vertebral arch at the back of the spinal column, the vertebral canal (the hollow inside the spinal column) is revealed. Starting from the first cervical vertebra (and moving down) below the sacrum, we can clearly observe the dura mater spinalis. See Figure (2-4)

This advanced level of anatomical observation was practiced by medical scientists in China over 2,000 years ago, as is evidenced by the text *Nan Jing*, Chapter 28 which says: "However, *Du mai* starts from the *Shu* point at the bottom of the spine, merges into the spinal column, goes upward to *Feng Fu*, and enters into the brain." Once the exposed dura mater spinalis and arachnoid are cut and removed, we see that the *Sui* (known to modern anatomy as bone marrow) almost fills the entire space inside the spinal column. See Figure (2-5).

This statement verifies that as early as 2,000 years ago Chinese doctors conducted anatomic experiments. They discovered the marrow in the hollow inside the spinal column, as well as the sea of *Jingmai*, the governor of *Jingmai*, and the pivot of *Jingmai*.

Medical scientists in ancient China discovered that *Jingmai* in the human body merge into the hollow inside the spinal column, forming the sea of *Jingmai*. They also described the way in which *Jingmai* converged and how the *Du mai* was located in the hollow inside the spinal column. They likewise knew how the *Jingmai* of the entire body are governed, and they conducted extensive medical research, achieving great advances in the field of medicine. Note, for example, in the text *Zhen Jiu Jia Yi Jing Chapter 4 - Zhen Dao*, it is said: "Crossings of *Jie*, 365 junctions. For those who know the essence, one sentence is enough; those who do not know talk pointlessly and endlessly. The so-called *Jie* are places where *Shen Qi* travels in and out, they are not skin, muscles, tendons, bones." This passage describes in detail (what we know today) as the anterolateral and posterolateral spinal tracts and neurofilments. The front and rear roots allow the free transmissions of information in and out, and are not made of skin, muscles, tendons, or bones.

There is no record of when the above discussion was first completed. We only know that it was written many centuries ago, and that through the years scholars have argued about it but never reached a consensus. Later on, a great medical expert summarized it accurately by saying that "The so-called *Jie* are places where *Shen Qi* travels in and out; they are not skin, muscles, tendons, bones." Although these are only the words of one expert, they has been widely accepted and passed down through the centuries.

The author of *Ling Shu Chapter 1 - Nine Needles and Twelve Source Points* is not only an expert practitioner of piercing *Jingmai* to treat disease; he is also a great theorist in the research of *Jingmai*. He was familiar with and mastered an understanding of *Jingmai* in the hollows inside the spinal column, and he knew the value and significance of this

Spinal Cord and Nerve Structures

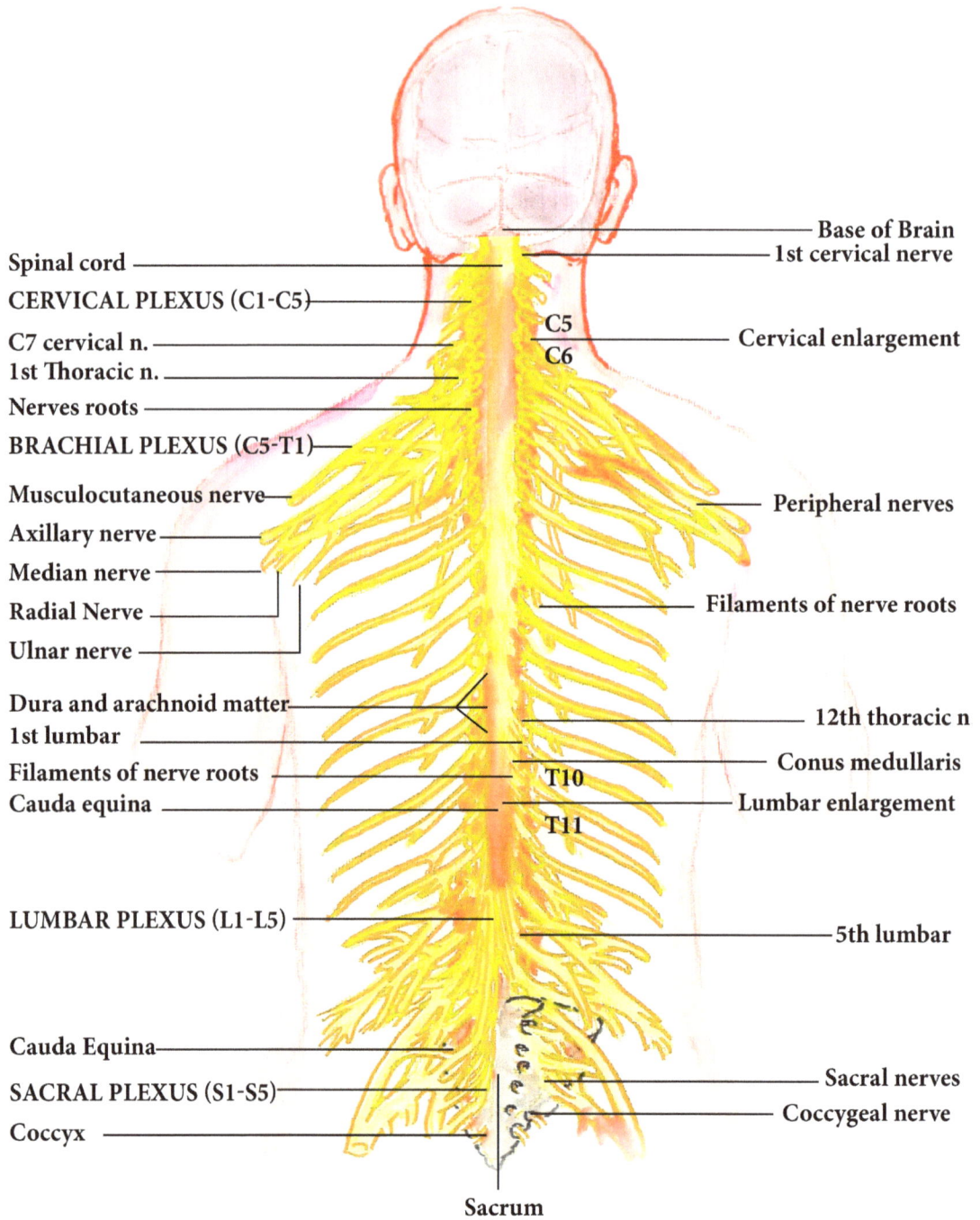

Spinal cord

CERVICAL PLEXUS (C1-C5)

C7 cervical n.

1st Thoracic n.

Nerves roots

BRACHIAL PLEXUS (C5-T1)

Musculocutaneous nerve

Axillary nerve

Median nerve

Radial Nerve

Ulnar nerve

Dura and arachnoid matter

1st lumbar

Filaments of nerve roots

Cauda equina

LUMBAR PLEXUS (L1-L5)

Cauda Equina

SACRAL PLEXUS (S1-S5)

Coccyx

Base of Brain

1st cervical nerve

C5

C6

Cervical enlargement

Peripheral nerves

Filaments of nerve roots

12th thoracic n

Conus medullaris

T10

Lumbar enlargement

T11

5th lumbar

Sacral nerves

Coccygeal nerve

Sacrum

[2-4 and 5]

finding. He boldly pioneered a method for describing *Jingmai* by starting (research in) *Jingmai* in the hollows inside the spinal column. His consequent achievements revealed the *Jingmai* to be a holistic system that deals with death and life, and that regulates the balance of the entire body. His work laid the scientific and theoretic foundations for using fine needles to pierce *Jingmai*, and for treating diseases through (energy balance and) adjustment.

Section 2.2 - Somatic *Jingmai*

Somatic *Jingmais* and their treatment using fine needles is of great clincial importance in Chinese acupuncture.

Because somatic *Jingmai* are pierced directly by fine needles, medical experts pay special attention to the somatic *Jingmai* and study them in depth. *Due* to differences of opinion, perspectives and methods vary. Here I can only summarize the research that has been done on the subject in anatomy, physiology and clinical acupuncture.

I. Research in the fields of anatomy and physiological experimentation.

Medical experts in ancient China were not only great clinical practitioners; they were astute and observant students of *Jingmai* as well. They initiated early research on *Jingmai* and made substantial achievements with their efforts. Before *Jiu Juan* there was a specialized book known as *Jingmai*. Evidence (for this) can be found in the preface of the ancient text *Zhen Jiu Jia Yi Jing* which declares that "*Jiu Juan* is the original version of the book *Jingmai*; its meaning is profound, and it is difficult to understand." *Ling Shu Chapter 1 - Nine Needles and Twelve Source Points* also pays special attention to somatic *Jingmai*. The following is a summary of related contents from this book.

(A) Crossings of Jie, 365 Hui

Zhen Jiu Jia Yi Jing Chapter 4 - Zhen Dao says: "Crossings of *Jie*, 365 hui." This sentence presents a conclusive summary of somatic *Jingmai* research. The so-called Crossings of *Jie* are the junctions of *Jie* and *Jingmai*. "Fan 365 hui" refers to the 365 junctions (also to *Jingmai* located deep inside the 365 acupuncture points) on the human body. These crossings are formed at multiple junctions of the *Jie* of *Jingmai*, a unique observation made via careful study of anatomy. Over the centuries, future generations did not understand this statement, and there were many contradictory and conflicting opinions concerning its true meaning. In the *Zhen Jiu Jia Yi Jing Chapter 4 - Zhen Dao*, it says: ". . . . For those who know the essence, one sentence is enough; those who do not know talk pointlessly and endlessly." *Ling Shu Chapter 1 - Nine Needles and Twelve Source Points* used this sentence to describe somatic *Jingmai*. Again, future generations did not comprehend the importance of this fact and the text was ignored for centuries.

(B) *Shun Ni Chu Ru Zhi Hui*

Ling Shu Chapter 1 - Nine Needles and Twelve Source Points pioneered a new way of describing somatic *Jingmai* as "Junctions where *Qi* flow and counter flow, exits and enters." By using "Junctions where *Qi* flow and counter flow, exits and enters" to express *Jingmai*, we know that the author of *Ling Shu Chapter 1 - Nine Needles and Twelve Source Points* was well acquainted with the fact that each somatic *Jingmai* can freely transmit information in and out (of itself). If he did not think this concept was accurate he would certainly not have included it in his book. There is no record in regard to what method was used by ancient scientists to test this theory.

Where do the somatic *Jingmais* join? Are there flows and counter flows, entrances and exits in *Jingmai*? These questions can only be answered through a study of anatomy and physiological functions. *Jingmais* in the hollow inside the spinal column are formed by *Jingmais* all over the body (at the points) where they merge together. It is found that *Jingmais* in the hollows inside the spinal column are somatic *Jingmais*.

If we consult an anatomical textbook on the subject of neurological anatomy, we find that the nerves that pass in and out of the spinal marrow are somatic nerves. These nerves are formed by multiple junctions of the anterolateral and posterolateral spinal tracts and neurofilaments. See Figures (2-6), (2-7), (2-8), (2-9), (2-10), (2-11), (2-12) and (2-13A&B).

The somatic nerves can transmit out-going motor information and in-coming sensory information. The fact that the structural purpose of the nerve junctions and their function is to transmit information in and out is consistent with the findings of *Jingmai* as described by ancient scientists. This convergence of old theory and new proves that the somatic nerves (peripheral nerves) identified in modern medicine are the same somatic *Jingmais* that were identified by ancient scientists.

Based on the above we know that the somatic nerves in the human body were first discovered 2,000 years ago by ancient Chinese scientists, and that this knowlege was used by Chinese doctors in their clinical practice. It was only many centuries later (during the time of the Renaissance) that the existence of the somatic nerves was discovered in the West.

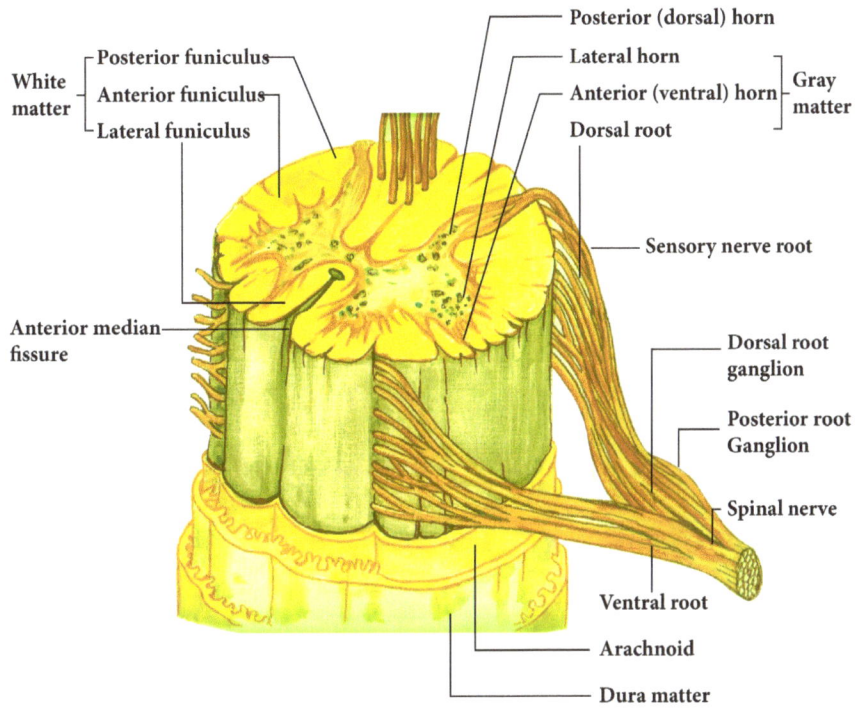

White matter
- Posterior funiculus
- Anterior funiculus
- Lateral funiculus

- Posterior (dorsal) horn
- Lateral horn
- Anterior (ventral) horn
- Dorsal root

Gray matter

Anterior median fissure

Sensory nerve root

Dorsal root ganglion

Posterior root Ganglion

Spinal nerve

Ventral root

Arachnoid

Dura matter

[2-6] Nerve Root Ganglion

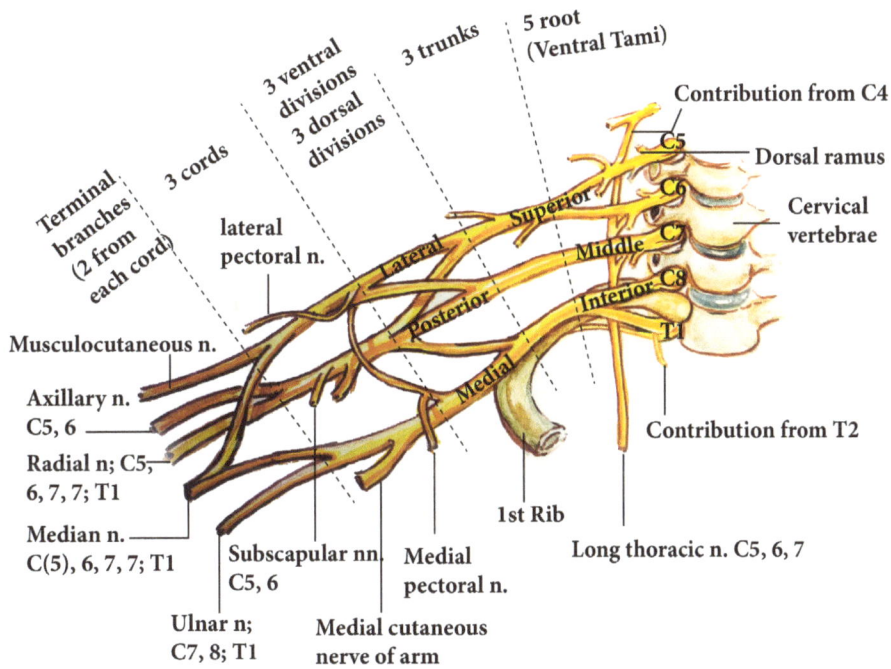

5 root (Ventral Tami)

3 trunks

3 ventral divisions
3 dorsal divisions

3 cords

Terminal branches (2 from each cord)

Contribution from C4

C5

Dorsal ramus

Cervical vertebrae

C6

Superior

C7

Middle

C8

Inferior

T1

lateral pectoral n.

Lateral

Posterior

Medial

Musculocutaneous n.

Axillary n. C5, 6

Radial n; C5, 6, 7, 7; T1

Median n. C(5), 6, 7, 7; T1

Subscapular nn. C5, 6

Medial pectoral n.

1st Rib

Contribution from T2

Long thoracic n. C5, 6, 7

Ulnar n; C7, 8; T1

Medial cutaneous nerve of arm

[2-7] Right Brachial Plexus

43

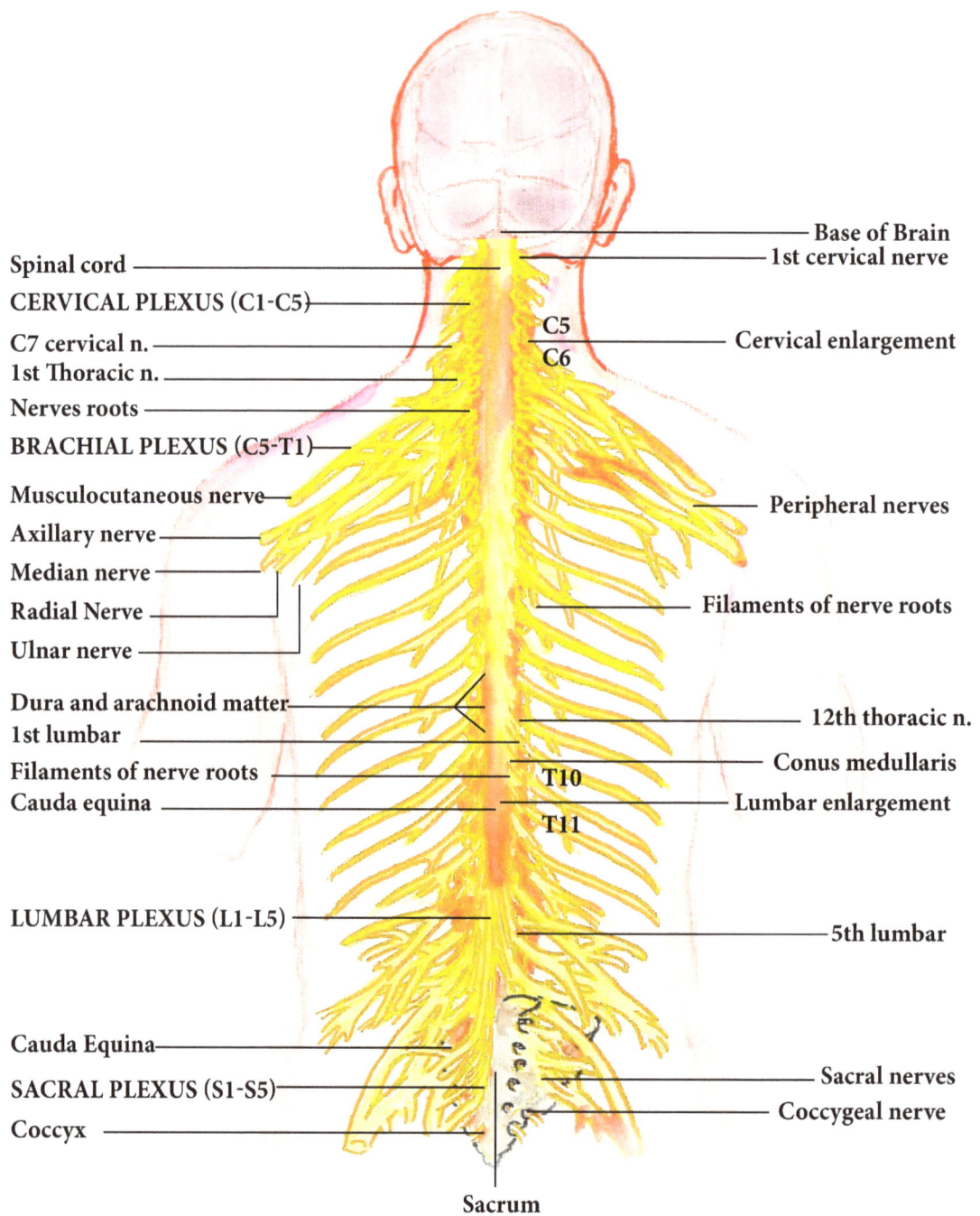

Base of Brain
1st cervical nerve

Spinal cord

CERVICAL PLEXUS (C1-C5)

C5

C6

Cervical enlargement

C7 cervical n.

1st Thoracic n.

Nerves roots

BRACHIAL PLEXUS (C5-T1)

Musculocutaneous nerve

Peripheral nerves

Axillary nerve

Median nerve

Radial Nerve

Filaments of nerve roots

Ulnar nerve

Dura and arachnoid matter

12th thoracic n.

1st lumbar

Filaments of nerve roots

Conus medullaris

T10

Cauda equina

Lumbar enlargement

T11

LUMBAR PLEXUS (L1-L5)

5th lumbar

Cauda Equina

SACRAL PLEXUS (S1-S5)

Sacral nerves

Coccygeal nerve

Coccyx

Sacrum

[2-8] Spinal Cord and Nerve Structure

44

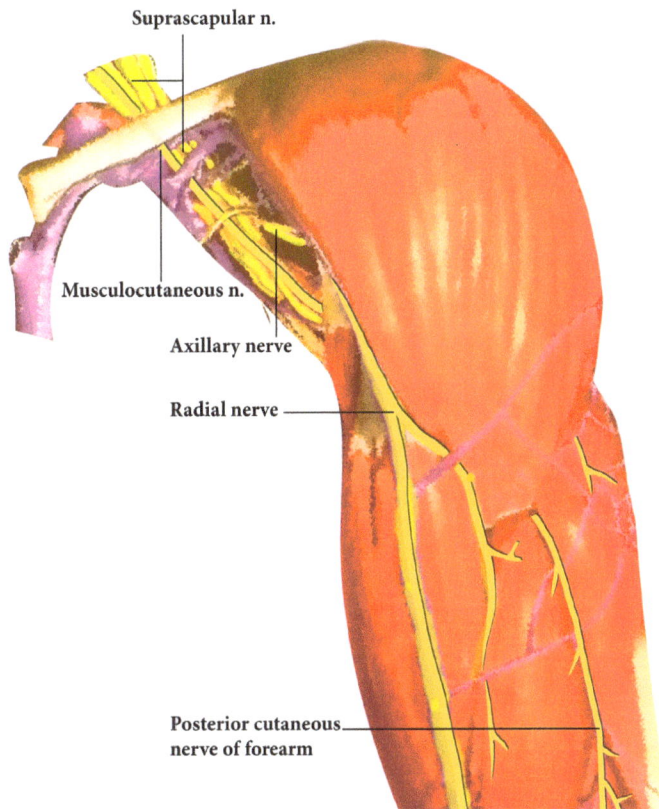

Suprascapular n.

Musculocutaneous n.

Axillary nerve

Radial nerve

Posterior cutaneous
nerve of forearm

[2-9] Scapular Axillary and Radial Nerve

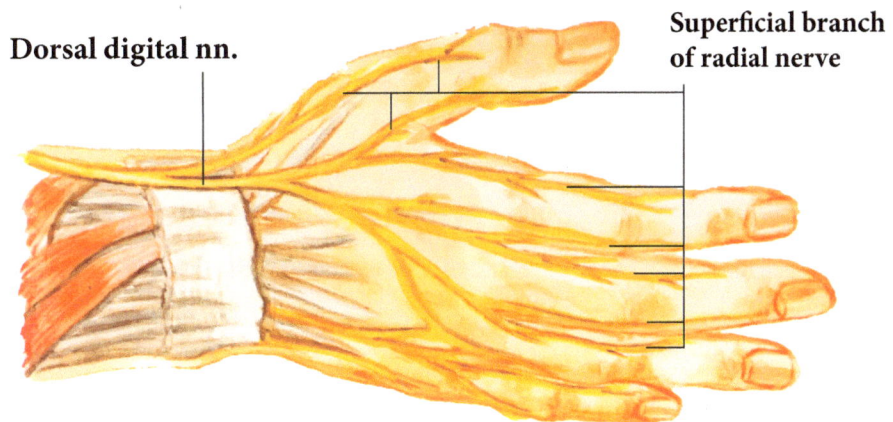

Dorsal digital nn.

Superficial branch
of radial nerve

[2-10] Nerve of Hand

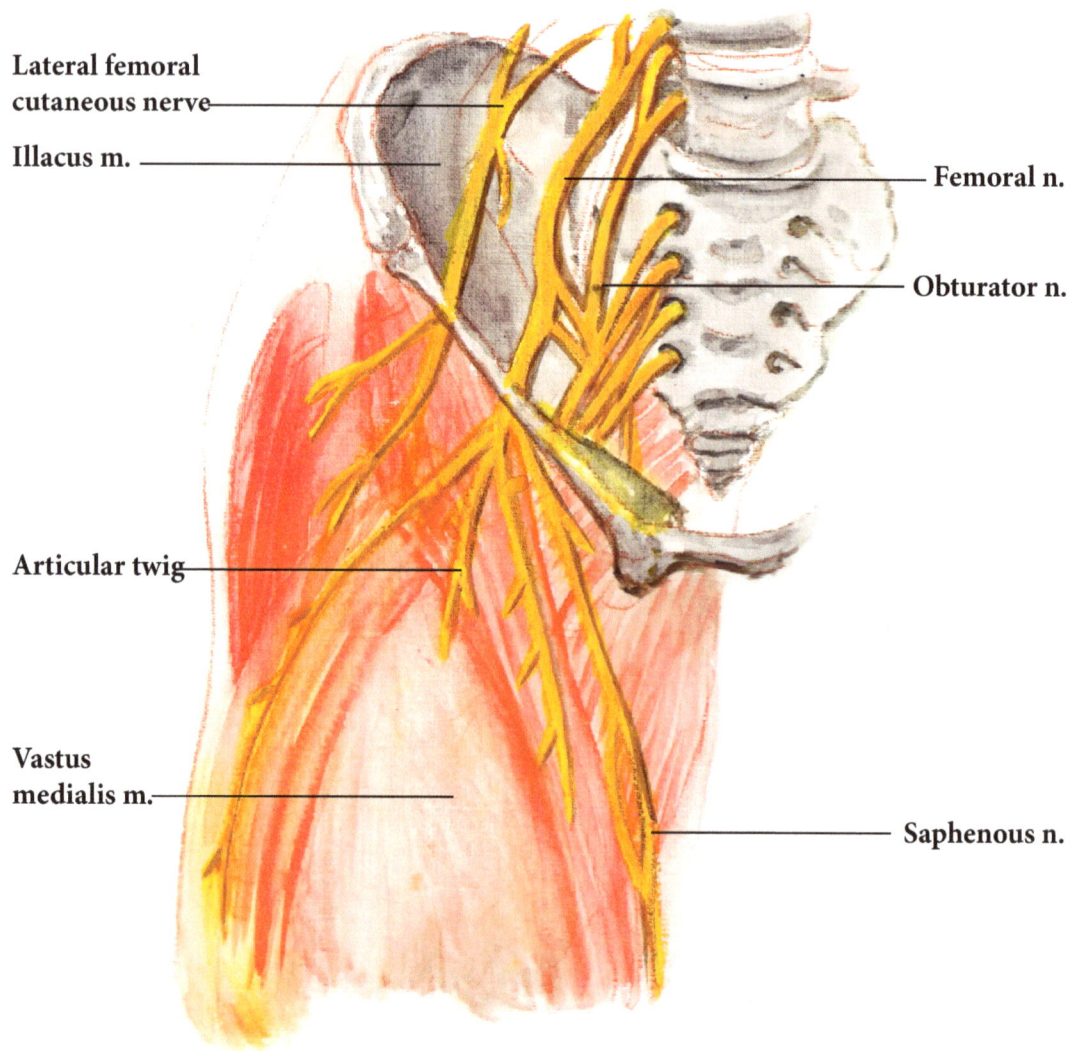

Lateral femoral cutaneous nerve

Illacus m.

Femoral n.

Obturator n.

Articular twig

Vastus medialis m.

Saphenous n.

[2-11] Femoral and Lateral Cutaneous Nerve

Common peroneal n.

Superficial
peroneal n.

Deep peroneal n.

Medial dorsal
cutaneous n.

Lateral dorsal
cutaneous n.

Saphenous n.

Medial
cutaneous
branches of
saphenous n.

Medial branch
of deep peroneal n.

Proper dorsal digital nn.

Sciatic nerve

Tibial nerve

Common peroneal n.

Crural
interosseous n.

Soleus m.

Medial calcaneal branch

Sural n.

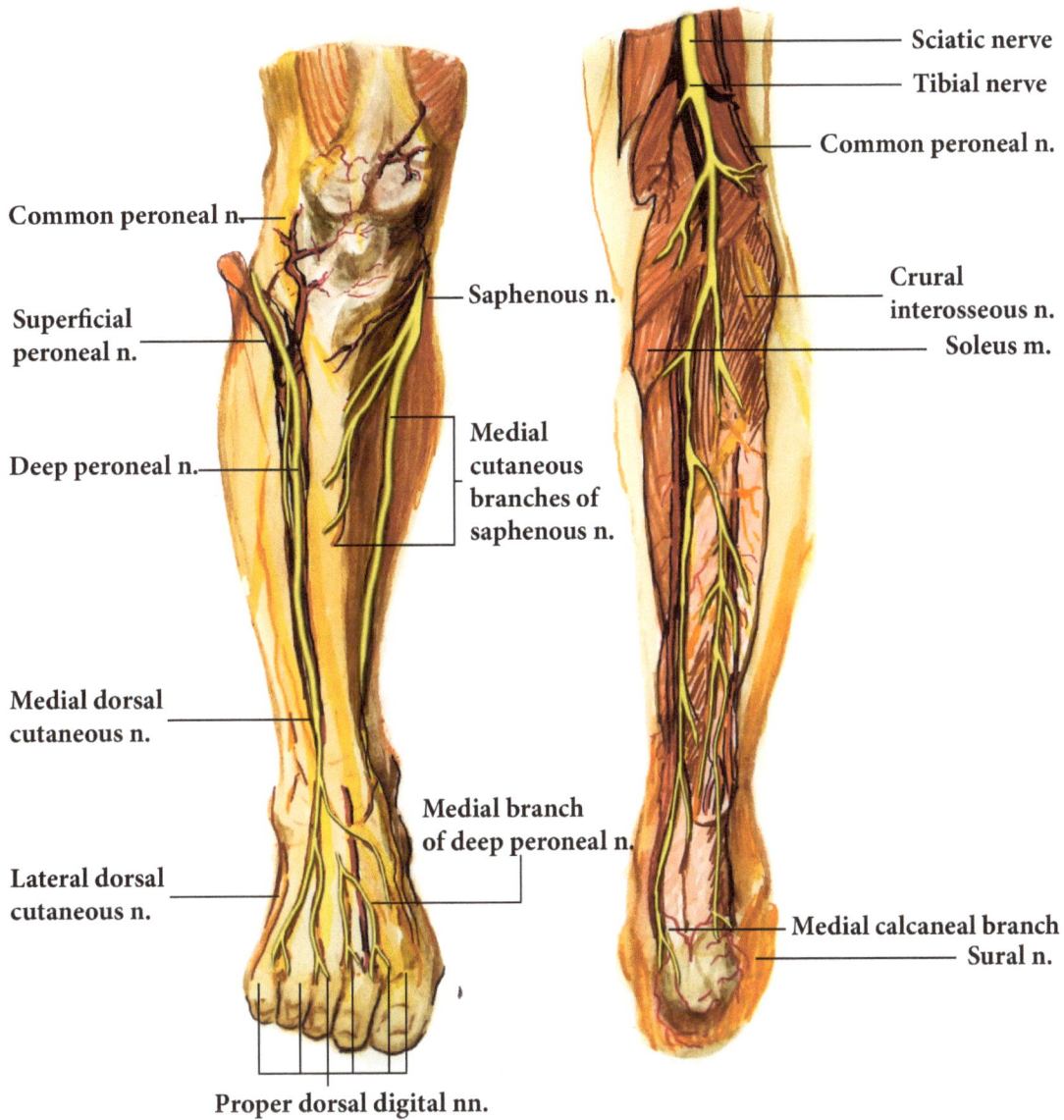

[2-12] Sciatic Tibial and Common Peroneal Nerves

47

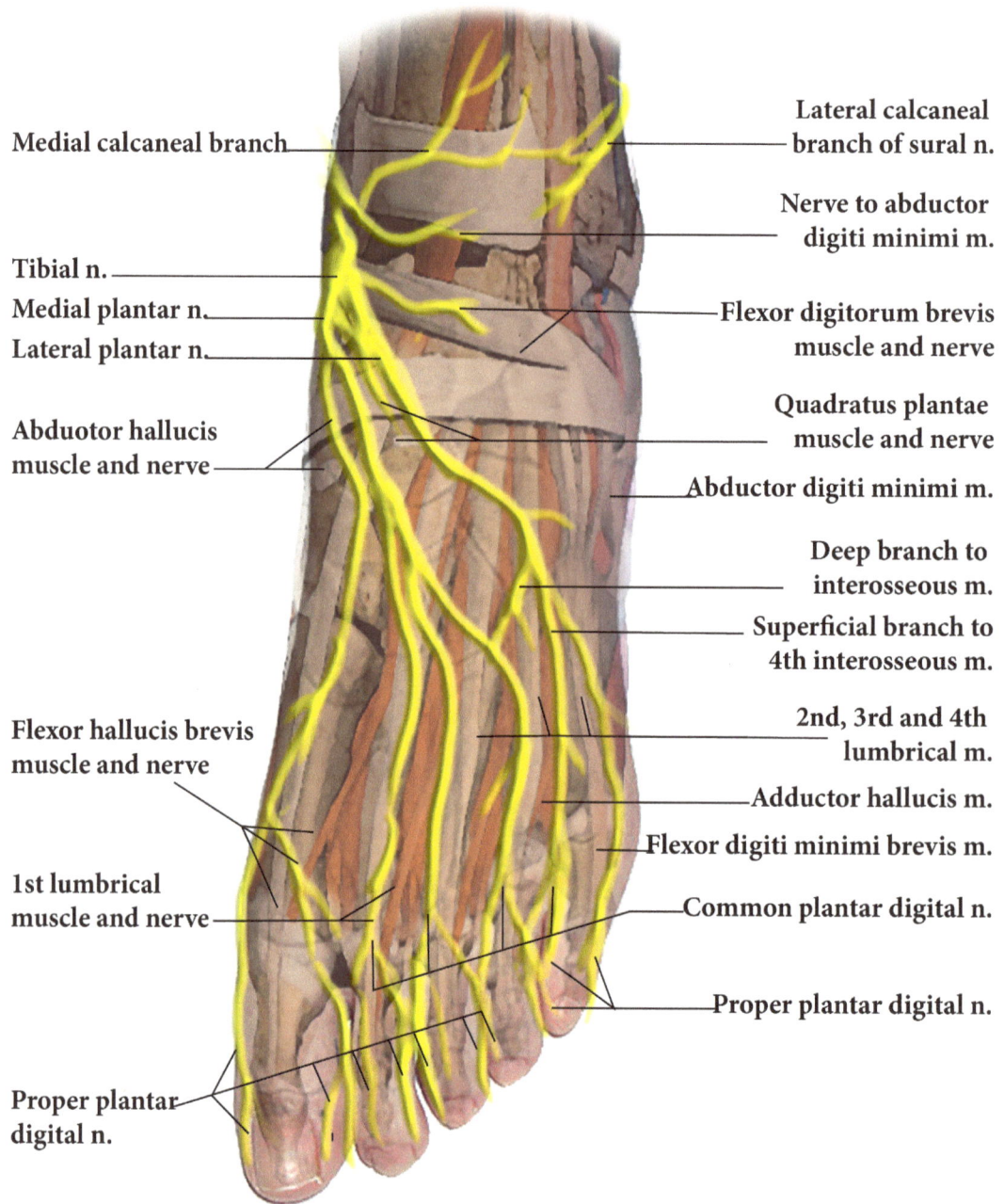

Medial calcaneal branch

Lateral calcaneal branch of sural n.

Nerve to abductor digiti minimi m.

Tibial n.

Medial plantar n.

Lateral plantar n.

Flexor digitorum brevis muscle and nerve

Quadratus plantae muscle and nerve

Abductor digiti minimi m.

Abduotor hallucis muscle and nerve

Deep branch to interosseous m.

Superficial branch to 4th interosseous m.

2nd, 3rd and 4th lumbrical m.

Flexor hallucis brevis muscle and nerve

Adductor hallucis m.

Flexor digiti minimi brevis m.

1st lumbrical muscle and nerve

Common plantar digital n.

Proper plantar digital n.

Proper plantar digital n.

[2-13A] Peroneal Nerve of Foot

48

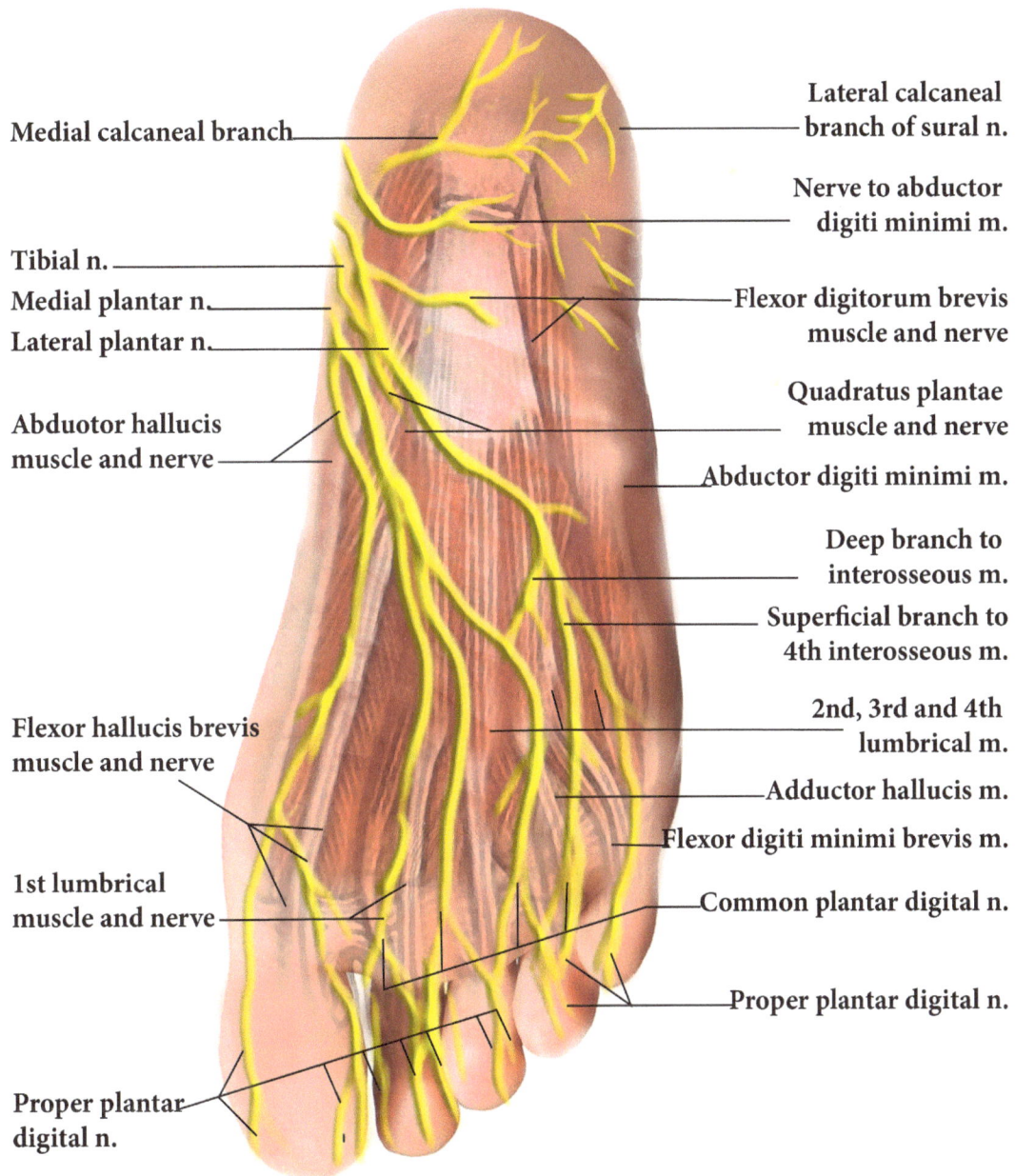

Medial calcaneal branch

Lateral calcaneal
branch of sural n.

Nerve to abductor
digiti minimi m.

Tibial n.

Medial plantar n.

Lateral plantar n.

Flexor digitorum brevis
muscle and nerve

Quadratus plantae
muscle and nerve

Abductor digiti minimi m.

Abduotor hallucis
muscle and nerve

Deep branch to
interosseous m.

Superficial branch to
4th interosseous m.

2nd, 3rd and 4th
lumbrical m.

Flexor hallucis brevis
muscle and nerve

Adductor hallucis m.

Flexor digiti minimi brevis m.

1st lumbrical
muscle and nerve

Common plantar digital n.

Proper plantar digital n.

Proper plantar
digital n.

[2-13B] Peroneal Nerve of Foot

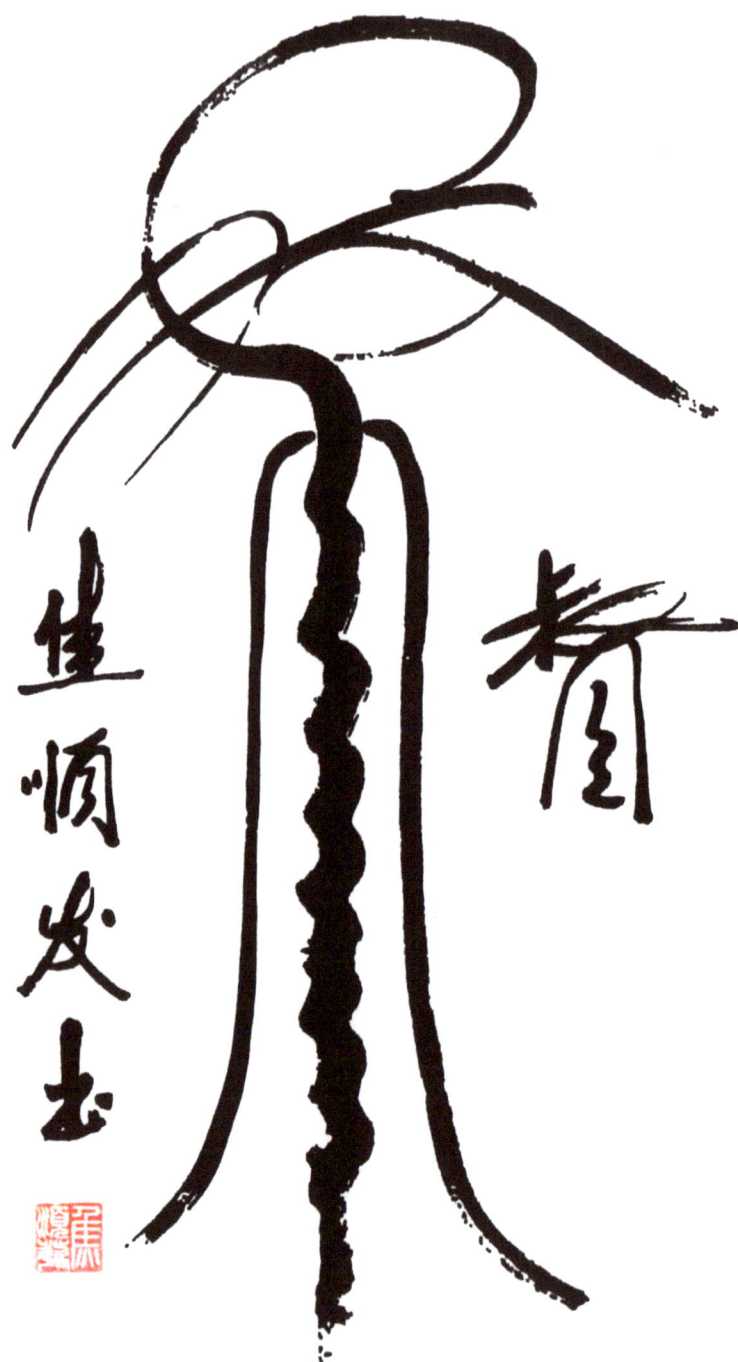

"DU MAI"
Calligraphy by Dr. Jiao

CHAPTER THREE

On Using Fine Needles To Pierce Jingmai

———

"Ling Shu Chapter 1 - Nine Needles and Twelve Source Points emphatically encourages the use of fine needles to treat disease, giving fine needle acupuncture a special purpose and mission. Since the time of its writing fine needles were widely used for piercing Jingmai to treat diseases.

Medical scientists in ancient China invented fine needles thousands of years ago and used them to pierce the Jingmais to treat diseases, thus proving the value of this treatment many times over. These early practitioners deserve to be congratulated!"

Ling Shu Chapter 1 - Nine Needles and Twelve Source Points advocates the use of fine needles to pierce *Jingmai*. The sentence "I want to use fine needles to open up its *Jingmai*" provides evidence for this statement.

If we read the sentence "using fine needles to pierce *Jingmai*" in a literal way it seems like a simple statement. But in fact (through the years) it has exerted enormous scientific influence on all branches of clinical Chinese acupuncture. Although Chinese acupuncturists began to use fine needles millennia ago, many medical experts did not understand their importance in piercing the *Jingmai*. They only knew that once they pierced certain acupoints distinct healing effects could be achieved. Later, after a long period of clinical practice and in-depth research, Chinese medical experts began to make certain important observations such as the fact that "(The doctor) must pierce the *Qi* point," "pierce the *Qi* point," "pierce *Shen*," and "pierce *Ji*." Those who planned, experimented, and wrote *Ling Shu Chapter 1 - Nine Needles and Twelve Source Points* carefully summarized all this past medical experience, and used it to inform their text.

The appearance of the statement "using fine needles to pierce *Jingmai*" launched this specific practice and led to a new era of medical treatment. From that time on China's use of fine needles to pierce *Jingmai* and treat disease rapidly developed in a scientific way. Unfortunately, future generations did not understand *Ling Shu Chapter 1 - Nine Needles and Twelve Source Points* as well as they should. The result was that a complete and full understanding of the *Jingmai* was ignored and largely forgotten. This was a tragedy for the future history of Chinese medicine. Therefore, (if we are to exploit its full value) we need to truly understand the meaning of the *Ling Shu*'s original text and express its ideas correctly in modern language (in order to fully profit from the wisdom of its authors). Only by so doing can we vigorously promote the ideas (of the masters who created it) and pass them on to posterity. The following interpretations are based on the meaning of the original text.

Section 3.1 - Fine Needles

By using fine needles to treat disease, and by observing the fact that patients tended to improve when treated this way, Chinese doctors thousands of years ago invented the art of fine needle acupuncture. Through the years fine needles were continuously improved in terms of their quality, width, and length. There is, however, no documented evidence regarding when fine needles actually first appeared, though it is estimated that they were in wide use as early as 3,500 years ago. *Ling Shu Chapter 1 - Nine Needles and Twelve Source Points* says: "*The Great Essentials* says: 'Slow then rapid is excess. Rapid then slow is deficiency.'" This statement offers evidence that fine needle acupuncture was in clinical use at a very early date.

Ling Shu Chapter 1 - Nine Needles and Twelve Source Points emphatically encourages the use of fine needles to treat disease, giving fine needle acupuncture a special purpose and mission. Since the time of its writing fine needles were widely used for piercing *Jingmai* to treat diseases.

Medical scientists in ancient China invented fine needles thousands of years ago and used them to pierce the *Jingmais* to treat diseases, thus proving the value of this treatment many times over. These early practitioners deserve to be congratulated!

The purpose of discussing fine needles is to understand (their use, function, and value) correctly. In the future, acupuncture *Jingmais* for treating disease will continue to use fine needles exclusively.

Section 3.2 - Holding Needles

The way to hold a needle is an important aspect of acupuncture *Jingmais*. The *Jingmais* can only be stimulated correctly if practitioners grip the needle in the proper way.

Ling Shu Chapter 1 - Nine Needles and Twelve Source Points says: "As for the way to hold a needle, holding it in a firm way is precious." The statement "holding it in a firm way is precious" does not imply that the firmer one grips a needle the better. It is saying that it is good to hold the needle firmly when piercing the body and *Jingmai*, but not to hold it too firmly. In truth, it is extremely difficult to explain how to master one's grip on a needle. One can only learn this art thoroughly through (long years of) clinical experience.

Section 3.3 - Pierce into the Skin

Using a fine needle to pierce the skin is the first step in applying *Jingmai* acupuncture. As a result, it is important (for the doctor) to practice piercing in an effective manner. There are two issues to be aware of in this regard. First, if we are to pierce the *Jingmai* accurately we must needle the point in the proper way. Second, we must pierce through the skin quickly in order to reduce the patient's pain.

Section 3.4 - The Direction of Piercing

When it comes to the direction of needling, *Ling Shu Chapter 1 - Nine Needles and Twelve Source Points* provides two descriptions:

I. Pierce perpendicularly

First, the sentence "*Zheng zhi zhi ci, wu zhen zuo you*" tells us to pierce perpendicularly and to not (incline the) needle to the left or right.

II. The direction that triggers the "arrival of Qi" is the correct direction

The direction that triggers the "arrival of *Qi*" is the correct direction. If *Qi* does not arrive the technique is incorrect. "When *Qi* goes away, it is called counter flow (*Ni*); when it arrives, it is called flow (*Shun*). When counter flow and flow are grasped, positive (healing) actions can be taken without (doubts or) questions" tells us that if the "arrival of *Qi*" occurs when pushing in a needle this means the direction of the needle is correct (a condition termed "*Shun*"). On the other hand, a direction that makes the "arrival of *Qi*" weak or causes it to dissipate is the wrong direction (which is termed "*Ni*"). As long as you know the *Shun* and *Ni*, pierce boldly with no more questions.

In clinical practice both the above methods are useful. We should use them flexibly according to the locations of the acupuncture point and the specific requirements of a given treatment. All in all, the number one choice of needle direction is the direction that best triggers the "arrival of *Qi*."

Section 3.5 - Pierce the *Jingmais*

Piercing *Jingmais* is the core technique that determines the success or failure of a treatment. Therefore, one must be familiar with this technique and practice it carefully. For better understanding, I will discuss it in three aspects.

I. Why should we pierce the Jingmai?

Ling Shu Chapter 1 - Nine Needles and Twelve Source Points considers piercing *Jingmai* to be the key to successful acupuncture treatment. The reason why acupuncture has achieved so much success over thousands of years is that it concentrates on piercing the *Jingmai*. Thus, we must seek to pierce the *Jingmai*. Here are some examples.

"A poor doctor only looks for the physical location of an acupoint, while a superior doctor seeks the spirit (*Shen*)." The "spirit" mentioned here is wondrous; it is "like a distinguished guest entering our door". This passage means that the inferior doctor knows only how to needle the physical location of the acupuncture points, while a superior doctor knows (how to find) the *Shen* in a point. That is, a superior doctor knows how to pierce the *Shen* in the *Jingmai* to treat disease. *Shen* is therefore a marvelous force. It is like an honorable guest who we welcome inside the *Jingmai*.

"A poor doctor only knows how to look for the physical joints (*Guan*) while the superior doctor knows how to find *Ji* – gate mechanismin the point. The movement of *Qi* never exceeds its space. When we observe it from the outside *Qi* activity appears tranquil in the space it occupies. It appears to have only a slight movement. Its coming cannot be met and its going cannot be followed or grasped. Those who understand the gate mechanism are able to pierce the points precisely without missing a hair's breadth. Those who do not understand gate mechanism will miss the timing of *Qi*. Piercing points in a random way is useless. Knowing where *Qi* is coming from and where it is going and timing of *Qi* to get the best result is important. This phenomenon is really wondrous. The poor doctor remains in the dark (about it), while the superior doctor knows all these (important facts). "

This passage means that the inferior doctor only knows how to apply needles to the physical points when treating disease, while the superior doctor knows how to find and pierce the *Ji* in these locations. Through anatomical and physiological experiment (including observation), it has been found that the movement of *Ji* never exceeds its space. *Ji* activity appears tranquil when we look at it from the outside. It only shows slight movement. But the activities going on within *Ji* are swift and delicate, transmitting information in and out. This phenomenon is difficult to detect with the naked eye. Those doctors who understand the essence of *Ji* will pierce it precisely; those who do not understand the essence of *Ji* will find (the *Ji* in the point) difficult to locate and pierce. By knowing the coming and going of *Ji* one can achieve the anticipated (healing) goal. This is a marvelous fact; an inferior doctor cannot see (into the essence of needling practice); only a superior doctor knows (what to do).

II. How do we decide whether the Jingmai is pierced?

Somatic *Jingmais* are located deep in the body. We cannot see them, nor can we see whether or not the needle has pierced them accurately. Ancient Chinese medical experts described the experience and insights they attained through clinical practice and the needling of the *Jingmai*. These are summarized as follows:

1. When we push the needle into the acupuncture point, if the resistance at the tip of the needle suddenly grows stronger this pressure means that the *Jingmai* is pierced. Otherwise the *Jingmai* is not pierced. (The important point is to sense when the resistance grows stronger)

Ling Shu Chapter 1 - Nine Needles and Twelve Source Points says: "*The Great Essentials* says: 'Slow then rapid is excess. Rapid then slow is deficiency.'" The meaning of this statement is that when we push a needle into an acupuncture point and the resistance at the tip of the needle suddenly becomes strong this means it is "firm" and that the needle has successfully pierced the *Jingmai*. On the other hand, if there is little or no resistance at the tip of the needle this indicates that the needle is still in a state of "emptiness." This condition of emptiness is called "Xu" and means that the *Jingmai* is not pierced. This feeling in the needle is very unique. It manifests as a sudden increase of resistance rather than the (even) resistance encountered as the needle slides in. This feeling, referred to as "wan chen," often occurs when the needle reaches the tendons and bones. When we experience this sensation we should withdraw the needle a small amount, change direction, and pierce again. *The Great Essentials* is an ancient text and its words prove that the above information was understood and put into practice long ago.

2. Once the "arrival of *Qi* (De *Qi*) occurs, it proves that the *Jingmai* is pierced."
Ling Shu Chapter 1 - Nine Needles and Twelve Source Points says: "(if you) pierce and *Qi* does not arrive, do not ask how many times (you have pieced); (if you) pierce and *Qi* arrives, remove the needle and (perform) no more piercing." The meaning of this passage is that if the "arrival of *Qi*" does not occur when piercing, keep piercing and do not ask

how many times (you must continue) to pierce. Once the "arrival of *Qi*" occurs remove the needle and stop piercing.

The essence of this passage is that we must seek to trigger *Qi Zhi* (the arrival of *Qi*) when practicing acupuncture *Ling Shu Chapter 1 - Nine Needles and Twelve Source Points* uses this passage to show that *Qi Zhi* signals the fact that *Jingmai* has been pierced. This description is of great significance. The understanding of acupuncture advanced considerably due to the practice of *Qi Zhi* and it remains very valuable (up to today).

The occurrence of *Qi Zhi* is a very important sign. It signifies that *Jingmai* has been pierced, and it foretells that relatively good (healing) results can now be expected. *Ling Shu Chapter 1 - Nine Needles and Twelve Source Points* tells us that: "The essence of needling is that once *Qi* arrives there is a (healing) response. This response appears quickly in the way that a sudden wind blows away the clouds and the sky becomes clear and blue. This is the complete *Tao* of needling. This is the evidence."

III. Piercing the Jingmai should be done in a moderate way
Ling Shu Chapter 1 - Nine Needles and Twelve Yuan-Source Points suggests that acupuncturists should not only pierce *Jingmai*, but that they should practice needling with extreme moderation. Medical experts in ancient China accumulated a great deal of clinical experience when practicing acupuncture. *Ling Shu Chapter 1 - Nine Needles and Twelve Yuan-Source Points* affirms (the validity) of these experiences and the need for stimulating the *Jingmai* in a moderate way.

Ling Shu Chapter 1 - Nine Needles and Twelve Yuan-Source Points says: "For those who practice acupuncture, (treat) deficiency by filling, excess by draining, chronic stagnation by eliminating and over abundance of evil *Qi* by withdrawing." This passage means that for those who practice acupuncture, if there is emptiness one should fill it. If there is fullness one should drain it. When the needle encounters "wan chen" (a situation where the tip of the needle reaches the tendons and bones), one should remove the needle. If the patient experiences severe shivering, numbness, or pain when the needle pierces the *Jingmai* (which is called "*Xie Shen*" accoding to ancient experts), one should weaken it. The original purpose of this text is to describe the reactions that can occur during acupuncture treatment and the specific solutions for these reactions. *Ling Shu Chapter 1 - Nine Needles and Twelve Yuan-Source Points* considers that these methods can be used to adjust the intensity of piercing *Jingmai*, and to achieve optimal and appropriate treatment. "Drain is called Ying and tonify is called 'follow.'" This is a classical statement that refers to adjusting the intensity of *Qi Zhi*.

To sum up, *Ling Shu Chapter 1 - Nine Needles and Twelve Yuan-Source Points* suggests that one should try to acupuncture *Jingmai* and that one should be moderate (in so doing). Generally speaking, when using acupuncturing *Jingmai* it should be obvious when *Qi Zhi* (arrival of *Qi*) occurs, but the sensation of its arrival should not be too strong. The best and most appropriate degree of *Qi Zhi* is when it is bearable for the patient. That said, to practice this method really well is not an easy task. One can only do so by reflecting continuously and by taking note of one's experiences in clinical practice. According to *Nine Needles and Twelve Source Points*, care must be taken in moderation when needling the *Jingmai*. In general, moderate "arrival of *Qi*" is ideal. Many acupuncturists attempt to trigger obvious "arrival of *Qi*" during treatment, but this arrival should not be so strong that the patient cannot tolerate it. (All in all, therefore) the above are mere words, but what really needs to be done in these circumstances is not an easy thing (to explain) or do. Only by intense clinical practice and repeated summary (and research) can the practice of *Jingmai* needling be mastered.

To sum up, the technique of using fine needles to acupuncture *Jingmai* as advocated and described by *Nine Needles and Twelve Source Points* is extremely important (in the practice of medicine). It has enormous scientific value and has made enormous contributions to Chinese acupuncture. We must understand this method correctly, take it seriously, promote it vigorously, and pass it on devotedly to future generations.

Epilogue

"Acupuncture somatic *Jingmai* to treat diseases" is the most distinctive healing feature of Chinese acupuncture.

The initiation of "Acupuncture somatic *Jingmai* to treat diseases" is a great pioneering work and has contributed significant research to Chinese medicine. It is the invention of Chinese medical experts, but it is also the achievement of world medical science.

Jiao Shun Fa
March 18, 2007

"Unique healing effect" offers a great competitive advantage in the Chinese art of acupuncture *Jingmai* for treating diseases.

Acupuncture *Jingmai* as invented by Chinese doctors treats various ailments all over the body and exerts unique healing effects on certain dieseases. As far as we know, no other medical treatment method can match (or surpass) it.

Jiao Shun Fa
March 18, 2007

As summarized and advocated by the ancient text *Ling Shu Chapter 1 - Nine Needles and Twelve Yuan-Source Points*, using fine needles to acupuncture *Jingmai* marks the maturity and high point of Chinese acupuncture's attempts to treat disease. It is the most significant research method that has ever evolved from Chinese acupuncture treatment.

Jiao Shun Fa
March 18, 2007

The method of using fine needles to acupuncture *Jingmai* and treat disease, as pioneered and advocated by the ancient text *Ling Shu Chapter 1 - Nine Needles and Twelve Yuan-Source Points* offers us a marvelous technique that is based on sound scientific theory and unique healing effects. As long as we understand this method correctly and consider it in a serious light, it will be like a towering tree (for all medical practitioners to see), standing tall in the forest of world medical science.

Jiao Shun Fa
March 18, 2007

Statements offered in the ancient text *Ling Shu Chapter 1 - Nine Needles and Twelve Yuan-Source Points* represent the core of *Ling Shu* and the essence of Chinese acupuncture treatment. It has great scientific value and practical significance. We must promote it vigorously and pass it on (to future generations) seriously.

Jiao Shun Fa
March 18, 2007

In short, as I read the *Nine Needles and Twelve Yuan-Source Points* I was filled with so much excitement, admiration, and inspiration that I cannot express my true esteem in ordinary words.

Jiao Shun Fa
March 18, 2007

道通古今 鍼

焦顺发

"The *Dao* of Acupuncture Throughout The Past And Present"
Calligraphy by Dr. Jiao

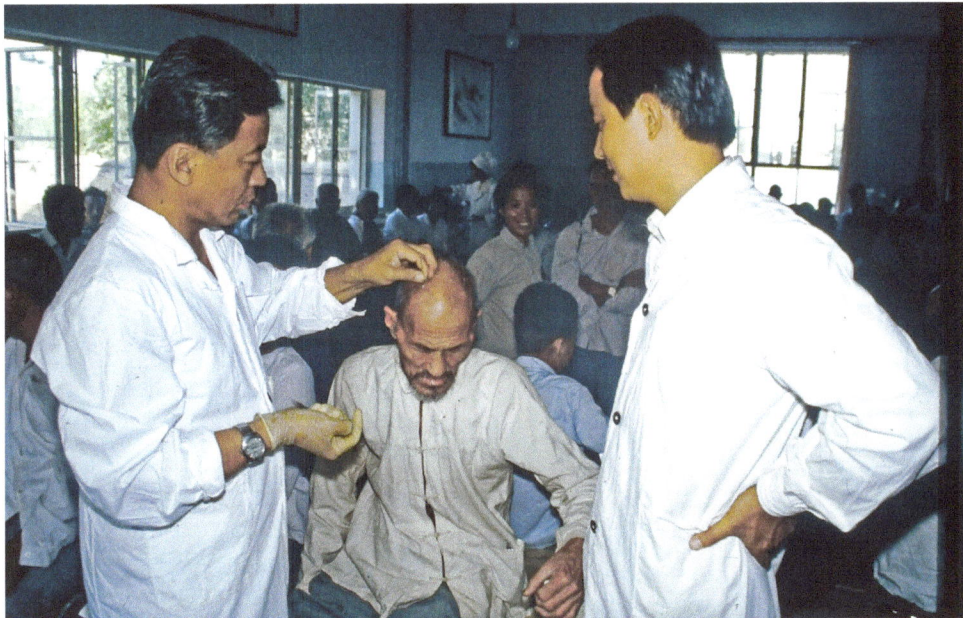

Dr. Jiao and Dr. Chan, Head Acupuncture Institute, Shanxi, China, 1983.

Dr. Tsoi Nam Chan has been a special friend and student of mine for almost 40 years. He is a gifted practitioner of the healing arts, as well as a master artist and calligrapher in the classical Chinese tradition. He is able to see and understand the connection between all aspects of life, which is evident in both his paintings and his approach to medicine. For Dr. Chan, treatment is more than just inserting needles; it is an all-encompassing art form that includes elements of *Qi Gong, Tai Qi, Feng Shui*, calligraphy, poetry, science, and philosophy.

Dr. Chan, moreover, is well versed in Western therapeutics as well as traditional Chinese medicine, and comfortably bridges the gap between ancient and modern forms of healing. His command of the English language plays an important part in his ability to translate deeply esoteric Chinese medical theories into clear English. For almost 30 years, his office located in New York City next to the United Nations has been filled with a healing spirit, as well as many interesting works of art. His patients comprised of people from all walks of life including foreign dignitaries, artists, celebrities and CEO's of Fortune Five Hundred companies.

Dr. Chan can truly comprehends the depth and nature of my theories, and is able to offer critical feedback and valuable advice. I am fortunate to know him as a friend, a colleague with whom I can discuss and share ideas, and as an intermediary through whom I can express important new interpretations of ancient wisdom in a way that is practical, logical and understandable. In addition to his help in translating, I would like to thank him for his designs and illustrations throughout this book.   ~ Dr. Jiao Shun Fa

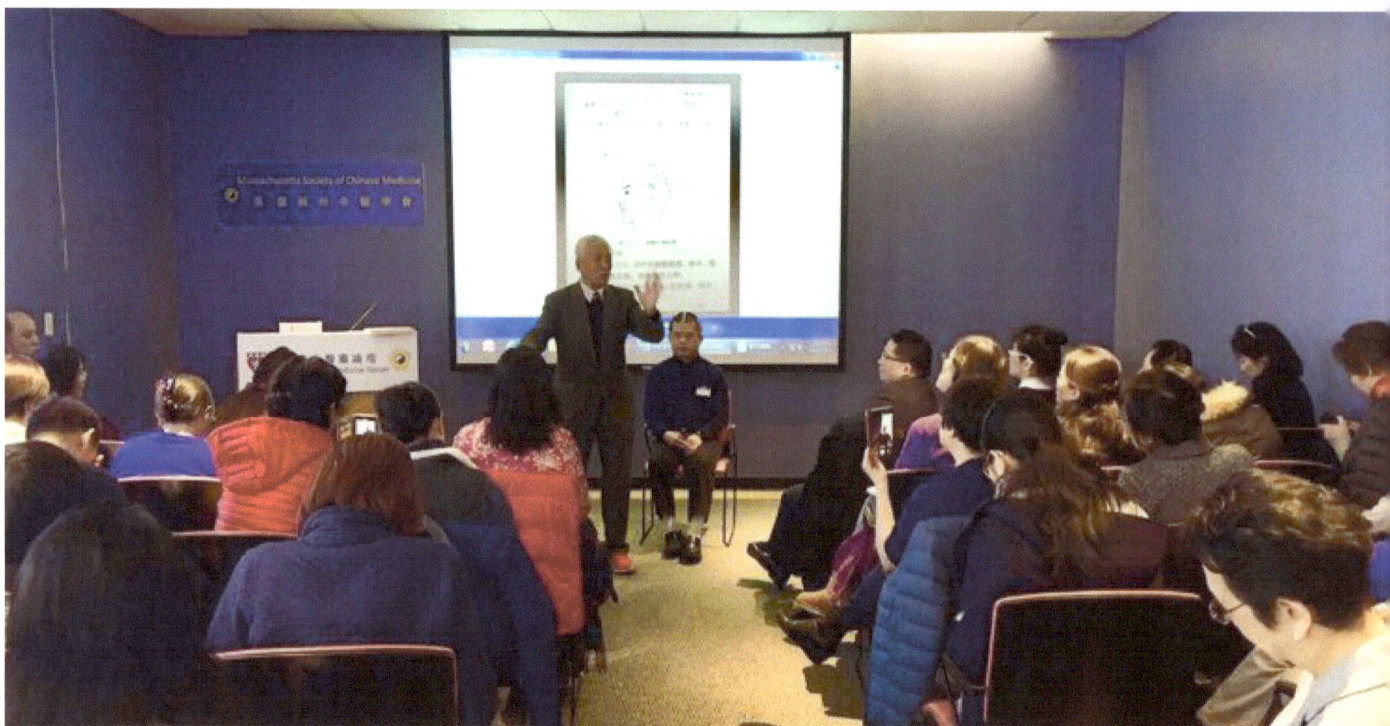
Harvard University, March, 2018.

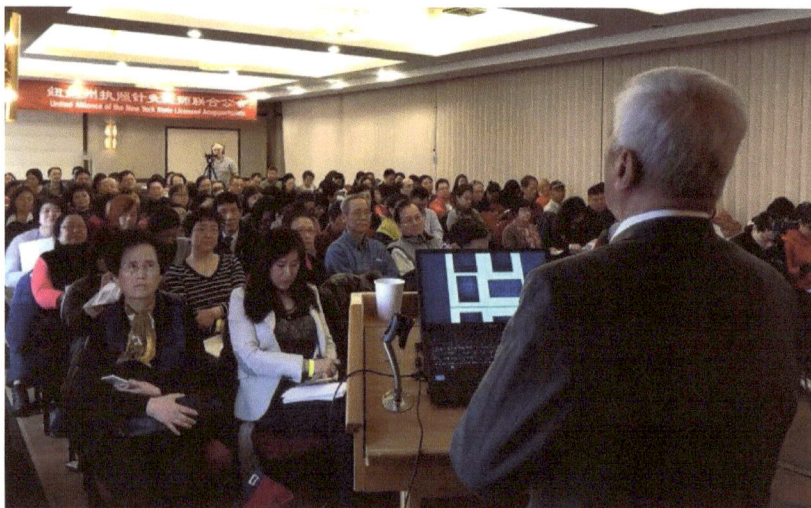
New York, March, 2018.

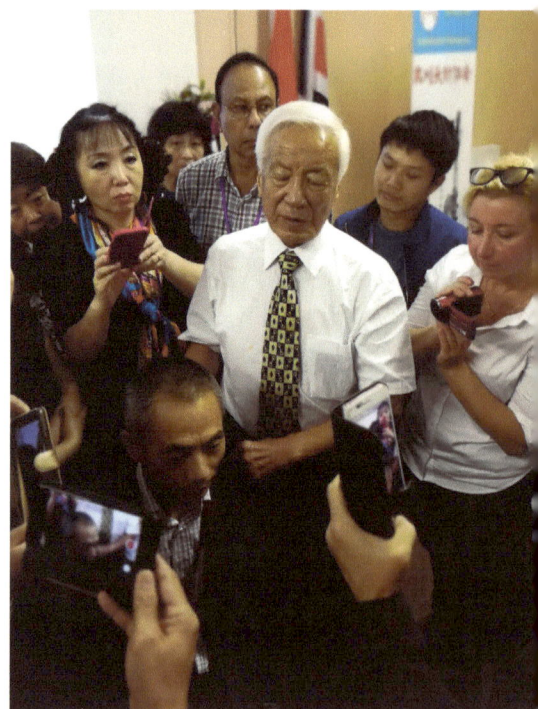
Manchester City, Germany, August, 2018.

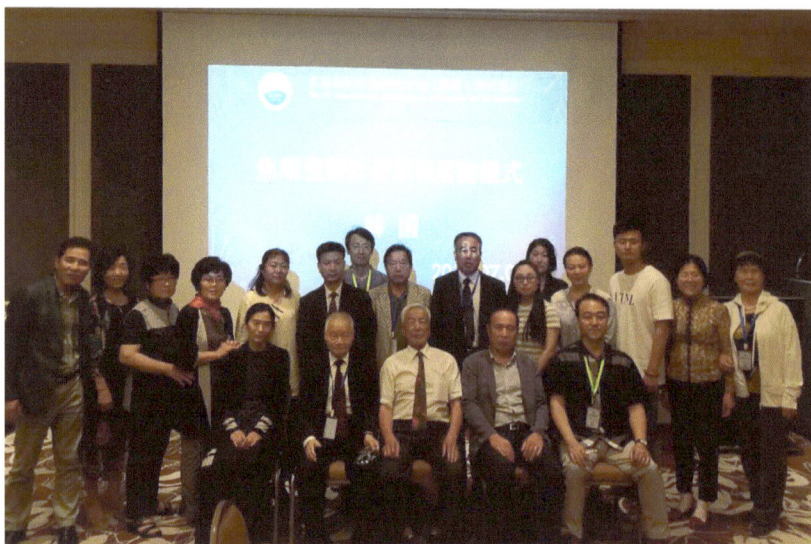
Jeju Island, South Korea, April, 2018.

Dr. Jiao has been teaching acupuncture and his ne
theory all over the world for almost 50 years. He h
written many books, some of them are being taught
graduate schools of traditional Chinese Medicine.

The countries include: China, U.S.A., Russia, Japa
Korea, England, Germany, Italy, Belgium, Jierjisi Sita
Kazakhstan, Holland, Belgium and Thailand.